Low-Carb Diet

2 Manuscripts In 1 Book:

Dirty Keto Diet

Endomorph Diet

Thomas Rohmer

Dirty Keto Diet

Lose Weight and Get in Great Shape Without Following Strict Ketogenic Rules

Thomas Rohmer

Copyright © 2018
Thomas Rohmer All rights reserved.

No part of this publication may be reproduced, distributed, or
transmitted in any form or by any means, including photocopying, recording, or other electronic or mechanical methods, without the prior written permission and consent of the publisher, except in the in the case of brief quotations embodied in product reviews and certain other noncommercial uses permitted by copyright law.

Disclaimer:

This guide has been created for informational and reference purposes only. The author, publisher, and any other affiliated parties cannot be held in any way accountable for any personal injuries or damage allegedly resulting from the information contained herein, or from any misuse of such guidance. Although strict measures have been taken to provide accurate information, the parties involved with the creation and publication of this guide take no responsibility for any issues that may arise from alleged discrepancies contained herein. It is strongly recommended that you consult a physician, personal trainer, and nutritionist prior to commencing this or any other workout or diet plan. This guide is not a substitute for professional personal guidance from a qualified medical professional. If you feel pain or discomfort at any point during exercises contained herein, cease the activity immediately and seek medical guidance.

Before You Begin:

Get the Latest Scoop on the Most Cutting Edge Info on Health & Fitness!

As thanks for picking up this book, I'd love to offer you the chance to maximize your results by getting exclusive info on health and fitness.

You'll be the first to know when I publish new books, and you'll receive exclusive content on health and fitness that I only share with people on my list.

Simply visit the link directly below and get started on the path to the healthiest version of yourself today!

https://rohmerfitness.lpages.co/kindle-sign-up/

Table of Contents

Chapter 1: What is the Standard Ketogenic Diet?....9

Chapter 2: Caloric Intake and Macro Percentages on a Dirty Keto Diet..16

Chapter 3: Why Most Fail with Keto and What You Can Do to Be Different..23

Chapter 4: How to Overcome the Keto Flu..............49

Chapter 5: How to Eat Keto at Restaurants, Parties, or Other Social Events..56

Chapter 6: The Importance of Sleep and Why It Can Make or Break Your Success...................................66

Chapter 7: How to Meal Prep on a Ketogenic Diet..87

Chapter 8: Building Muscle on a Dirty Ketogenic Diet..98

Chapter 9: Frequently Asked Questions................104

Introduction

Obesity is at an all-time high in America. This shouldn't be the case considering that we now have access to more information than we ever did before.

We have access to the latest information in nutrition, exercise, and supplementation, yet things only seem to be getting worse. The problem comes down to two main things.

The first is that we're being fed the wrong information. Yes, having access to a lot of information is great, assuming it's beneficial information. Sadly, this isn't the case most of the time, which is what keeps most of us stuck where we're at.

For example, a supplement company may promote things that aren't the full truth about their product so that they can increase sales. People may buy that supplement with the hope that they can achieve a certain result, when in reality, the supplement won't work. It wasn't the person's fault; they were just being told the wrong information, which is why he or she isn't getting the desired result.

Other times, the information might be good and factual but way too hard for the average individual to stick with. For example, some diet plans severely limit what foods you can and can't eat.

There may very well be a lot of good information that exists about that diet, but it could be too hard for the average individual to stick with for a prolonged period of time. If you quit on a diet, then you don't have any chance of success. A diet is only good as long as you can keep on doing it.

This is why it's so important to not only have the right information but also the right plan. You need both in order to succeed.

The right information with the wrong plan will cause you to quit, and the wrong information with the right plan will cause you to make mistakes that will hold you back.

That's why I plan to change things with this book. I'm going to give you the right information and the right plan in order to help you succeed. The plan we're going to use is the dirty ketogenic diet.

This is going to give us more flexibility than the regular keto diet, which will help make it a long-term sustainable diet. Additionally, you're also going to learn the correct way to do the dirty keto diet.

The reason why I say this is because it can be easy to approach the dirty keto diet with the wrong mentality. If you approach it thinking you can eat whatever you want as long as you're not eating carbs, then you have a long road ahead of you.

Yes, the dirty keto diet is awesome because it allows you to eat certain foods you normally wouldn't be able to on a standard keto diet, but you have to do it in the right way. That's what you're going to learn how to do in this book.

You're going to learn the proper way to do the dirty keto diet so that you can continue doing it for a long time to come. In fact, my goal is to make things to where it doesn't even feel like a diet.

The process needs to be as effortless as possible in order to get the best results. Don't get me wrong, sacrifices will have to be made; losing weight isn't a walk in the park. However, that doesn't mean we need to make things harder on ourselves for no good reason.

The dirty keto diet can help you reach your goal bodyweight and stay there for good. All that's left is to learn the necessary information, but before we get into that, would you please consider leaving a review for this book if you enjoy it? Even just a few words will help other people know if the book is right for them.

Many thanks in advance!

Chapter 1: What is the Standard Ketogenic Diet?

Before I get into the ins and outs of the dirty keto diet, it's important to first understand what the regular ketogenic diet is. The ketogenic diet is a high fat, moderate protein, and low-carb diet.

It was first recommended in the 1920's to help patients with epilepsy control their seizures. When people first hear about the ketogenic diet and how much fat you eat, they're usually alarmed.

This should come as no surprise since we've been told most of our lives that fat is bad for you. It can take a while to break through that mindset even after you've started the ketogenic diet.

In fact, when a lot of people first start a keto diet, they don't eat as much fat as they should! Again, a lot of this has to do with the lies we've been told about fats.

Now the point of the ketogenic diet is to get our bodies to use fat as fuel instead of carbohydrates. That's why the fat intake is so high on a ketogenic diet.

Our bodies' first source of energy is glucose. We get glucose from the foods that we eat. However, if we eat a low amount of carbs, then our bodies will have to get the energy it needs to continue functioning from somewhere else.

That somewhere else is going to be our fat stores. When we use fat for fuel instead of sugar, our bodies are in a state known as ketosis.

This is the state you want to be in when you're on the ketogenic diet. The main point of the ketogenic diet is to get your body to use fat as its main energy source instead of carbs.

The thing you have to remember is that, even if your body does adapt to using fat for fuel, this doesn't mean that things will always stay that way. For example, if your body has adapted to using fat for fuel, you still can't go back to eating a high amount of carbs.

If you do that, then you'll get kicked out of ketosis and go back to using sugar for fuel. By default, your body's first source of energy will be glucose.

If the glucose is present, then your body will use that for fuel first. This is why you must be committed to keeping your carb intake extremely low when it comes to a ketogenic diet; otherwise, the keto diet won't work for you.

However, keeping your carbs low isn't the only thing you have to be committed to when it comes to the ketogenic diet. You also have to eat a high amount of fat and a moderate amount of protein.

The reason why you have to eat a high amount of fat is that it will cause your body to produce more ketone bodies. The ketone bodies are going to be your body's new main source of fuel rather than glucose.

If you're not going to eat enough fat, then you're not going to produce enough ketone bodies. Not only that but if you're not eating enough fat, then that means you're either eating too many carbs or too much protein.

Eating too many carbs is bad for obvious reasons—you'll get kicked out of ketosis and have to use up that glucose before you can even think about getting back into that state.

However, eating too much protein is bad as well. Right now, you might not see the harm in eating a near equal amount of protein and fat in your diet.

For example, what would be so bad about eating 50% of your total calories from fat, 45% of your calories from protein, and 5% from carbs? Why does fat have to be higher and protein lower on a ketogenic diet?

Isn't protein supposed to be good for you? Yes, protein is good for you. It's very satiating, and it's responsible for repairing tissue, growing tissue, among other things.

However, you have to be careful that you don't over-consume it. The reason for this is that your body only needs so much protein on a daily basis.

With that being the case, what happens if you consume too much protein? What happens to the excess protein your body doesn't need?

It'll actually get converted into glucose via a process known as gluconeogenesis. This means that eating too much protein can actually end up kicking you out of ketosis.

While it may not sound like a good thing right now, if gluconeogenesis kicks in, it is for a good reason. It allows your body to keep functioning.

If you ever found yourself in a difficult situation like our ancestors did quite often, then your body would still have a way to get the energy it needs to continue sustaining your life, all thanks to processes such as gluconeogenesis.

So yes, there's a specific reason why you're eating the amount of fat, protein, and carbs that you are. It's all designed to help get your body into a state of ketosis so that you can use fat for fuel instead of carbs.

How Does the Dirty Keto Diet Differ From a Regular Ketogenic Diet?

So now that you know more of what a regular keto diet consists of, how does that differ from a dirty ketogenic diet? On a dirty ketogenic diet, you're still going to be consuming a high amount of fat, a moderate amount of protein, and a low amount of carbs.

Your primary goal is to get and stay in a state of ketosis, just like you would for the regular keto diet. A dirty ketogenic diet does not mean that you get to eat a higher amount of carbs, because that would defeat the purpose of the diet.

Instead, the main difference is the kind of foods that you'll be eating. On a regular or strict ketogenic diet, most of the foods you eat will be wholesome, organic foods.

For example, you would consume lots of vegetables that are high in fiber, various nuts and seeds, and organic butter. This is not to say that you can't consume these types of foods on a dirty keto diet because you certainly can if you want.

With a dirty keto diet, you may incorporate things such as artificial sweeteners, processed foods, and foods that are lower in fiber into your diet. Not everything you eat will be processed, but the difference is that processed foods are allowed on a dirty ketogenic diet, whereas the are not allowed on a strict keto diet.

Later on, I'll share with you the correct way to go about balancing the amount of clean and unclean foods you should eat on the dirty keto diet. There's a right and a wrong way to go about doing it, and you definitely don't want to mess it up.

Following a dirty ketogenic diet doesn't mean that you're allowed to eat whatever junk food you want, whenever you want, simply because it's low in carbs. There still needs to be a proper balance in place.

The main benefit of doing a dirty ketogenic diet is that it offers you more flexibility in your diet plan. This makes it much easier to do for a prolonged period of time.

You have to go into the dirty keto diet expecting to do it for years and years to come. If you don't, then your results will only last for as long as you're on the diet.

Most people have the wrong mentality when it comes to dieting. They try different diet plans in the hope of a quick fix. After they lose some weight, people often go back to their old way of eating, and then eventually they start to gain the weight back.

A lot of the time, this can be due to the fact that the diet plan was too restrictive or hard to keep up with. With the dirty keto diet, you're giving yourself some room to incorporate more of your favorite food choices, which makes it better for long-term sustainability.

What is Lazy Keto?

Another version of the keto diet is known as the lazy keto diet. Lazy keto doesn't deal with whether or not you'll eat strictly processed foods. Instead, it has more to do with tracking and measuring the foods that you eat.

On a ketogenic diet, it's critical that you know you're getting the right amount of fat, protein, and carbs. If you don't eat enough fat, then you might not be able to get into ketosis.

If you eat too much protein, then that extra protein could get converted to carbs via gluconeogenesis and kick you out of ketosis. And finally, if you eat too many carbs, your body will continue to use sugar for energy instead of fat.

And if you have no idea of how much of each macro you're eating, then you're simply hoping for the best. For this reason, I don't recommend the lazy keto diet if you are new to the ketogenic lifestyle.

You're still familiarizing yourself with what foods are keto approved and which ones aren't. You're still learning where carbs can be hidden in foods.

The last thing you want to do is take your best guess as to whether or not you're heading in the right direction.

This is why you need to make sure you track every calorie and macro that you eat.

Don't worry, I'll show you exactly how to do that in a later chapter. And while I understand that this can be a pain in the neck, I promise that it's for your own good.

This will ensure that you're not wasting your time spinning your wheels. At the end of the day, you're following this diet plan because you want to get results.

Remember that you have to be diligent with the diet plan if you want to get those results. The good news is that you don't have to strictly track your calories and macros for the rest of your life.

As time goes on, you'll get better and better at knowing what foods you can and cannot eat. You'll know how many calories and macros certain foods contain.

This is a skill you'll acquire as time goes on. In the beginning though, you have to stay diligent with tracking your calories and macros. Unfortunately, there's no way of getting around this if you want to optimize your results and ensure that you're heading in the right direction.

Chapter 2: Caloric Intake and Macro Percentages on a Dirty Keto Diet

In this chapter, we're going to figure out exactly how many calories it is that you need to be eating every day. We're also going to figure out what percentage of each macro we'll be eating and then converting that into calories.

First though, it's important to understand how your body works in regards to weight loss.

How do you lose weight?

Every day, our bodies need energy. We get this energy from the foods that we eat.

Our bodies then take this energy and use it to fuel processes such as breathing and organ function. The exact amount of energy our bodies need to continue functioning is known as our resting metabolic rate.

For example, if someone burns off 1,800 calories a day, then his or her resting metabolic rate is 1,800 calories. What would happen if we were to eat more calories than our resting metabolic rate?

Our bodies would then store the excess energy as fat. And if we eat less than our bodies burn, then we'll use our stored fat for energy. For example:

Cindy's resting metabolic rate is 1,800 calories. Therefore:

- If Cindy eats more than 1,800 calories per day, she'll be in a caloric surplus and start to gain weight.
- If Cindy eats less than 1,800 calories per day, she'll start to lose weight.
- If Cindy eats right at 1,800 calories per day, then she'll neither gain nor lose weight.

The only way your body loses weight is by being in a caloric deficit. Even if you're on a ketogenic diet, you can still overeat on fat and not lose any weight.

This is why we want to make sure that we know how many calories it is that we need to eat. And even after you know that number, you still need to continue to track the amount of calories that you are eating.

Here's how you can figure out what your resting metabolic rate is:

Resting metabolic rate = Current bodyweight x13

For example, if Cindy currently weighs 138 pounds, she'll take 138 and multiply it by 13 to get 1,800 calories per day. If Cindy wants to lose weight, she needs to eat less than 1,800 calories per day.

The question becomes how large of a caloric deficit should you aim to create? If you create too large of a deficit, then it'll make the diet plan harder to sustain for the long-term.

Sure you'll get results fast, but you'll end up crashing and burning. On the other hand, you don't want to create too small of a deficit.

It'll be easy to maintain, but you won't be losing weight at any considerable pace. Therefore, the best way to go about things is to go in the middle of these two extremes.

You want to aim for around 1 pound of fat loss per week. That might not seem like a lot, but remember we're talking about pure fat loss here.

This will add up to make a much bigger difference than you think. Losing even 5 pounds of fat can have a profound impact on how you look, but imagine losing 52 pounds of fat in one year!

That would make a big difference. I want to mention that you're more than likely going to lose more than one pound per week when you first get started on the ketogenic diet.

This is mostly going to be water weight. The reason people lose a lot of water weight when they first get started is that for every gram of glycogen you eat, the body will also store 3-4 grams of water.

Now that you won't be consuming any more carbs, your body will also be getting rid of that extra stored water. And since water isn't massless, the number on the scale will go down.

Remember though, it's not water loss that we're after here. The main thing we care about is fat loss. So after you've been on the keto diet for a few weeks, the main goal is going to be losing 1 pound of fat per week.

And since there are 3,500 calories in one pound of fat (1), this means you need to create a cumulative weekly caloric deficit of 3,500 calories in order to burn one pound of fat per week.

If you take 3,500 and divide it by 7 days in the week, this comes out to a total of 500 calories per day. Therefore to lose one pound of fat per week, you need to create an average daily deficit of 500 calories. Here's how to factor that in with your resting metabolic rate, using Cindy as an example:

Resting metabolic rate = 1,800 calories

1,800-500 = 1,300

Therefore Cindy needs to eat 1,300 calories per day in order to burn one pound of fat per week.

Calories aren't the only thing we need to be concerned with. We also have to track the amount of fat, carbs, and protein that we consume as well. These are the macronutrient percentages that we're going to be consuming on this dirty ketogenic diet:

Fat: 75% of our total daily calories
Protein: 20% of our total daily calories
Carbs: 5% of our total daily calories

Here's how to factor these macro percentages into your daily caloric intake:

1,300x.75 = 975 calories from fat
1,300x.2 = 260 calories from protein
1,300x.05 = 65 calories from carbs

You can then determine the gram equivalent by doing the following, since there are 9 calories per gram of fat and 4 calories per gram of protein and carbohydrate:

975/9 = 108.33 grams of fat per day
260/4 = 65 grams of protein per day
65/4 = 16.25 grams of carbs per day

How to Track Your Calorie and Macro Percentages

The next thing you need to do once you've calculated your calories and macro percentages is to actually track them. The easiest way to go about doing this is to use an app on your smartphone.

Simply type in "macro calculator" or "calorie calculator" and download one that you like. Most of them have similar features so it's hard to go wrong.

Once you have an app, the next thing you want to do is log all of the calories that you eat in the app. Most of the apps have barcode scanners, allowing you to easily scan and log whatever it is that you eat automatically.

You can also type in the food that you're eating, and log the nutritional information that way as well. The one thing you will need to know is the portion size of the foods that you're eating.

This is where something such as a food scale will come in handy. You will be able to know exactly how much of a certain food you're eating so you can determine the proper amount of calories and macros contained in it.

Even though modern technology will make tracking your calories and macros much easier, it's still a skill that you'll get better with as time goes on. Initially, you must be patient with yourself.

Now there will also be some times where you're not going to know exactly how many calories a certain food contains. For example, you might be at a party where one of your friends made a special recipe, and you have no idea what any of the nutritional information is.

In cases such as these, you're simply going to take your best guess as to how many calories are contained in that food. Obviously, since you're on a keto diet, you first and foremost need to make sure that it doesn't contain carbs.

After that, you're going to have to eyeball and guess how many calories the dish contains. This isn't easy by any means, especially considering the fact that you won't know how much protein or fat the dish contains either.

All you can do is take your best guess and move on. Do whatever you can to try and figure out the caloric and macro content of the dish.

Ultimately though, if you can't find that out, then you'll have to take your best guess. This can get you into trouble, as most people go about the eyeball test the wrong way.

They tend to underestimate the number of calories they eat. You don't want to do this because that can cause you to overeat.

For example, if your friend's dish contained 500 calories per serving and you estimated that it contained 300 calories, then you'll end up eating an extra 200 calories that you shouldn't have.

That's why it's much better to overestimate how many calories are contained in the foods you're unsure of. In this case, it'd be much better to estimate that the dish contained 700 calories even though in reality it only contained 500.

Sure you're still overshooting, but at least now you'll eat 200 fewer calories than you were supposed to at the end of the day.

This will still allow you to be in a caloric deficit, meaning you won't lose any progress as you work towards your weight loss goals.

For the most part though, most of the things you eat will be easy to track and measure. As time goes on, you'll easily be able to track the meals that you regularly eat because you'll already know the nutritional information.

It's just a matter of being patient with yourself as you get used to tracking your calories and macros. It can be a tedious thing to do at first, but it's well worth it to know that you're on the right track!

Chapter 3: Why Most Fail with Keto and What You Can Do to Be Different

It shouldn't come as a surprise that most people aren't successful when it comes to dieting. This holds true for the ketogenic diet.

Most people who start a ketogenic diet ultimately won't be successful with it for the long-term. And if we're being honest, long-term results are the only thing that matter.

If you lose 20 pounds on the ketogenic diet, and then you gain it all back 2 months later, what good did it do you? In this chapter, you're going to learn why it is that most people fail when it comes to dieting, and what you can do to ensure that you'll be different.

The Typical Dieting Mindset

Most people fail before a diet plan even begins. This can be for one of two main reasons—either the diet plan is setting people up for failure, or the person going on the diet has the wrong mentality.

Many of the mainstream diets are terrible, and they set people up to fail right from the start. An example of this would be something like a crash diet where the dieter would only be eating 500 calories per day.

This isn't going to end well for the person on the diet and rebound weight gain is going to occur. The other problem that often causes failure is the mindset of the individual.

Many people start a diet with the hope of a quick fix. They want to lose weight as fast as possible, but they don't have much of a plan for what they'll do once they lose the weight. Impatience is the real issue here.

You didn't gain all of the excess weight overnight, and you can't expect to lose it all overnight either. That's why it's better to think of things as a lifestyle change instead of a diet.

When someone says that he or she is going on a diet, this means that eventually that person will go off that diet. Whenever that happens, he or she will start to gain the weight back.

The phrase "going on a diet" implies the short-term. It means doing something miserable for as long as you can handle it.

When you finally can't take it anymore, you quit and go back to your old way of eating. Instead of doing this, think of things in terms of a lifestyle change.

This phrase implies permanent change for the rest of your life. This has a much more powerful impact on your subconscious mind.

Now making something a lifestyle change doesn't mean eating 500 calories a day and calling that a lifestyle change instead of a diet. It means doing things in a way that makes whatever nutrition plan you're doing sustainable for the long haul.

And in the case of the dirty ketogenic diet, that's exactly what we're doing. On the strict ketogenic diet for example, if you drank a diet soda, you'd technically be breaking the rules of the diet.

This could make you feel like a failure and make you want to quit the plan. However, this would still be allowed on the dirty keto diet, making it much easier to follow.

If drinking a diet soda every now and again helps you keep your sanity and allows you to keep on marching forward, then by all means do it. That's just one example of course, but implementing a proper lifestyle change comes down to striking a balance between structure and flexibility.

If a nutrition plan is too rigid, then you won't be able to keep up with it for years and years to come. On the other hand, if you have too much flexibility, then you might not end up with enough guidelines that'll allow you to get results.

Your diet plan could look similar to your old way of eating simply because there are no rules for your new nutrition plan. Thankfully, the dirty ketogenic diet will allow you to have a nice balance between structure and flexibility.

You have rules for certain things that you're not going to be able to eat (such as carbohydrates). Yet, these rules aren't so strict that it feels like you're in prison.

Throughout the rest of this book, I'm still going to be using the word diet in the normal sense that you're used to. From now on though, when you hear the word diet, I don't want you to think about it in the short-term 'get quick results' way that most people do.

I want you to view it more as a long-term permanent change because that's the only way that you'll truly be successful.

How to Stop Emotional Eating

Another thing that holds a lot of people back when on the ketogenic diet is the 'emotional eating' habit, which is when you eat to distract yourself from a certain feeling or emotion, as opposed to eating because you are truly hungry.

This can be especially dangerous on the ketogenic diet because you may binge eat on something that contains a lot of carbs, which means you'll get kicked out of ketosis. And most of the time "comfort foods" such as potato chips and ice cream are some of the first things people reach for when they eat out of emotion.

These foods are high in fat and sugar, which take energy from our nervous system and transfer it to the digestive system. This is why eating these kinds of foods can literally make us feel temporarily numb to whatever emotion it is that we're feeling.

And once someone gets kicked out of ketosis, it can be a slippery slope for a lot of people from that point forward. Once you've eaten a lot of carbs, it's easy to say to yourself, "Well I already got kicked out of ketosis, I might as well eat whatever it is that I want!"

The thing about this is that one meal can turn into one day, which turns into 2 days, which turns into a week or longer without ever getting back on track. That's why it's so important to recognize when you're eating out of emotion instead of hunger.

The reality is that we eat food to nourish our bodies and to get energy. We don't need to eat to cope with a certain emotion that we're feeling.

There are other ways to cope that don't involve eating too many calories. So what should you do if you know you eat out of emotion sometimes?

The first thing and most important thing that you can do is to be aware. You want to first and foremost notice what emotion it is that you're feeling whenever you binge eat some ice cream, for example.

When you catch yourself eating something like ice cream, ask yourself "What emotion am I trying to run away from right now?" It could be sadness, anger, fear, or something else.

Most of us think that it's not okay to experience saddening emotions. The truth is that it is perfectly fine and normal to feel these things.

In fact, we wouldn't know what happiness truly felt like if we weren't able to compare it to sadness. While it is okay to feel these things at times, it's not okay to bury the emotion and try to forget about it.

It will resurface, and it needs to be addressed. You could have experienced something as a child, and when something triggers you, it brings back that emotion you felt as a kid.

For example, a woman might fear that a man will never truly love her. Maybe she feels this way because her father was never around in her life growing up as a child.

These feelings might carry over into her adult life. When she starts dating, someone might text her and cancel the date on her and not give much of a reason why.

She'll feel like her date canceled because no man will ever love her. The reality is that her date could've gotten busy at work or something else came up, and he had to cancel.

However, that doesn't matter because that's not the story the woman is telling herself. Instead, she might go home and binge eat to help cope with her feelings of sadness.

Soon afterwards though, she'll feel even worse than before because she knows that she ate a lot of something she shouldn't have, and now she feels unloved, guilty, and bloated.

This can cause more feelings of sadness and hopelessness, which can lead to more emotional eating. This is why the cycle can be so vicious and hard to break through.

So in this case, what should this woman do to break out of her habit of emotional eating? She should first recognize that she wants to binge eat.

Then she needs to ask herself, why am I feeling the way that I am right now? She would then come to realize that it's because her date canceled on her.

This is a good start, but it's not deep enough. She needs to ask herself why it is that she's so upset about the situation.

Yes, it's understandable to be upset, but why is she going into a complete tailspin over this? She needs to think of moments from her past and see if there's any reason why she might be feeling this way.

At that point, she might realize that she never really felt loved by her father. This could be the reason why she's feeling insecure when someone cancels a date.

Figuring this out is very powerful. She can now break the cycle because of this awareness. It wouldn't be enough to simply be aware though.

You must find a way to be able to handle the emotion instead of trying to bury it away. In this case, communication would be the key.

She would need to make sure that she gets a good explanation for why her date canceled and see if they can reschedule. She can't assume that her date canceled because no one will ever love her.

She has to challenge those original assumptions and see if there's any truth to them. In this case, just because her father wasn't around doesn't mean that there won't be a good guy for her to date.

Even if someone would completely stand her up, that wouldn't mean it was her fault. The guy could simply be a jerk who has his own problems he's dealing with.

This is what she would need to understand and recognize so that she can feel confident in who she is as a person. Another example might be someone who eats because he's bored.

In this case, he would need to figure out when and where it is that he eats out of boredom. He may realize that he eats when he watches television at home.

If nothing good is on at the moment, he might eat as a way to make up for the boring shows. If this is the case, then he needs to find something different to do other than watching TV.

Maybe he could start a game night with his friends, read a book, or learn a new skill. Essentially, he would need to do something else that would help distract him and help him keep his mind off of food.

Even if he's aware of the problem, that might not be enough. As soon as he starts to get bored again, he may reach for the potato chips without even realizing it. The best thing he can do is stay as busy as possible or else the cycle will keep repeating itself.

What Can You Do to Become More Aware?

This information might sound great, but how can you become more aware if most of the time you don't catch yourself emotionally eating? Thankfully, there are a couple of different things that you can do.

The first one is to start asking yourself *why* you ate after every meal you eat. For example, if you normally eat dinner at 7:00, then you'll know you ate because that's when you usually eat.

However, if you got a snack at the vending machine, then ask yourself why you ate that candy bar. Were you actually hungry? Or are you trying to distract yourself from your work?

You have to ask yourself why after every meal you eat for the sake of consistency. This will help you make it into a habit, making it more likely that you'll be able to catch yourself when you're eating out of emotion.

The next thing that you can do is set an alarm for the end of the day. When the alarm goes off, think about what all you ate for the day, and why it was that you ate those things.

Did the soap opera really make the ice cream taste that much better, or are you stressed out at work? Did you get fast food because you truly wanted it, or because you're worn out and tired after a long day?

Finally, the most effective thing you can do is keep a food log. Basically, you'll log everything that you eat and also write what emotion you were feeling when you ate that food.

For example, if you ate some ice cream, you would log that you ate ice cream at 9:00 and that you were feeling sad. This is how you'll be able to become more aware of whether or not you're emotionally eating.

How to Stop Binge Eating

The next thing that trips a lot of people up on the ketogenic diet is binge eating. The reason why this happens is because people may have the wrong mentality.

For example, the person might be at a work event where lots of delicious non-ketogenic foods are being served. If the person eats something that isn't ketogenic, then he might feel that he can eat whatever he wants now because he already ruined his diet plan.

This is especially true on the ketogenic diet. Once someone eats more carbs than he should have, then the person feels that he might as well eat whatever he wants since he's already been kicked out of ketosis.

The thing is though, once you get kicked out of ketosis, you might not continue following the diet because of how long it'll take you to get back into ketosis. The next day you might wake up and think, "Well I'm already out of ketosis so I might as well eat how I please today."

If you do that for another day, it only makes it that much harder to get back on track with the ketogenic diet. And before you know it, it could be weeks or months since you've last eaten keto.

Binge eating is a problem with any diet plan; however, it's especially something that you'll want to be aware of when you're on the ketogenic diet. Being in ketosis is the main point of the ketogenic diet.

While it makes sense that people would eat however they please when they are out of ketosis, it's important to resist the temptation. Like I mentioned earlier, this could create a vicious cycle where long amounts of time go by before you get back on track. Think of it like working out in the gym.

Let's say you have a schedule to workout 5 days a week after you get off work. On Wednesday, you're really tired, and you decide to go home instead of going to the gym.

Then when Thursday rolls around, do you think it's going to be easier or harder to go to the gym after work? It's going to be a little bit harder because you skipped yesterday.

And if you skip your workout on Thursday, then it's going to be that much easier to skip on Friday. Then the next thing you know it'll be weeks before you go back.

Now consider the opposite scenario. If you workout on Monday, you will create momentum that will make it slightly easier for you to go on Tuesday. Then if you workout on Tuesday, that will make it a little bit easier to go on Wednesday.

The same is true for the ketogenic diet. Every day that you do the ketogenic diet will make it that much easier for you to continue doing it.

Each day you don't follow the ketogenic diet will make it that much harder to get back into it. Thinking of this ahead of time will help you out.

For example, let's say you've been following the dirty ketogenic diet for 3 weeks without any problems. Then you're at an office party and you're surrounded by a bunch of delicious carbs.

Before you decide to eat anything you know you shouldn't, you can think about how you'll be breaking your streak of 3 weeks. You can then think about how hard it'll be to get back in the groove of eating a ketogenic diet and ask yourself if that moment of glory will truly be worth it.

In most cases, it won't be. It'll likely bring up feelings of guilt and potentially lead to you spiraling out of control and eating whatever you want. Not only that, but these cravings of certain carbs that you may have will come and go.

As time goes on, you won't crave these foods like you used to. However, let's say you did eat something you feel you shouldn't have.

What should you do in these cases? For example, let's say you ate a brownie and ice cream at the party.

First and foremost, you must stop the bleeding. Think about what you do when you get a cut. Do you say to yourself, "I'm bleeding! I guess I might as well keep on bleeding until I've bled a good amount."

No, of course you don't say that. Instead, when you start bleeding, you apply pressure and a bandage in order to stop the bleeding.

You don't want things to get any worse than they already are. Sadly, when it comes to binge eating, most people have the kind of attitude as if they should keep bleeding!

If you ate something high in carbs, then you might as well splurge and eat to your heart's content. Of course, that is the wrong attitude to have.

Instead, you're much better off stopping the bleeding. If you ate a brownie and ice cream, then leave it at that.

Don't use getting kicked out of ketosis as an excuse to eat whatever you want for the rest of the day. Remember that the more carbs you eat, the longer it's going to take to burn off those carbs, thus making it that much longer for you to get back into ketosis.

Even if you ate something that kicked you out of ketosis, you can stop the bleeding and get back in it that much sooner if you don't binge eat everything in sight. Continuing to eat will only make the feelings of guilt and regret that much harder to overcome.

This leads me to my next point, which is that you have to understand that mistakes will happen. You're human, and you're not perfect. Going into this dirty ketogenic diet, the idea is to limit your carbohydrate intake to 5% of your total calories.

Doing that every single day for the rest of your life would mean that you did things perfectly. However, there are very few people who would be able to diligently follow a diet plan 100% of the time.

There might be moments where you eat too many carbs. That's okay as long as you pick yourself back up and keep on moving forward.

The only thing that can stop you is you. If you make a mistake and eat too many carbs, you have one of two choices.

You can admit to yourself that you're human and things like this will happen at times, or you can quit and go back to your old habits of eating.

If you choose the latter, then you're guaranteed to not get any more results. Embracing the fact that things won't always go smoothly will make it easier to move on from mistakes whenever they do happen.

Most people don't do that though. They tell themselves that things have to go perfectly. This creates an image in your mind that you'll never slip up and eat something that you're not supposed to.

When you do eat something you're not supposed to, then you're not acting in a way that's consistent with what you told yourself. This is what leads to feelings of guilt, frustration, and ultimately leads to you quitting.

Then you'll go back to your old eating habits because it's easy to stay perfect when you're eating whatever it is that you please. Instead, if you tell yourself that you will slip up at times, then you'll still be consistent with your beliefs when something does go wrong. This'll make it much easier to move past it.

How to Use Implementation Intention to Increase Your Chances of Success

What typically happens when people start a new diet or exercise plan? People say that they're going to do something, but then they struggle to actually do it.

Saying that you're going to do something and thinking about doing it usually isn't enough for people to be able to consistently follow through. This is where a technique known as implementation intention comes in handy.

Implementation intention is where you write down the conditions of completing a certain task. One study compared three different groups. The first group was told to follow an exercise routine for the next two weeks. The second group was told the same thing, and they were also shown videos about the benefits of exercise.

The final group was also told to exercise and watch the videos; in addition, the final group was told to write down by their own hand that they would exercise, including the specific time and place for when and where they would exercise.

The results didn't find much of a difference in exercise adherence between the first and second group. However, the third group was more than twice as likely to stick to the exercise plan in comparison to the other two groups (2).

Those are some pretty crazy results considering the fact that all you have to do is write a simple sentence. What makes writing that one sentence so powerful?

It comes down to something known as decision fatigue. We only have so much willpower to make decisions with. As the day goes on, our willpower starts to drain.

Once it's drained, your ability to start the things you know you should do (such as exercise or eating healthier) goes way down. In fact, it's even been said that the decision to workout takes more willpower than it does to actually do the workout itself.

This is why you'll see successful people wear the same thing every day. It allows them to not have to waste their precious deciding power on a trivial decision such as what to wear for the day.

Instead, they can save their willpower for much more important decisions later on in the day. With implementation intention, you're essentially doing the same thing as a successful businessman who wears the same thing every day.

You're already deciding ahead of time what it is that you're going to do when you're fresh. So how can you use implementation intention to increase your chances of success with the dirty ketogenic diet?

You can use it to plan out your meals ahead of time. For example, you could write down and say something along the lines of, "I eat three ketogenic meals at 8:00 a.m., 1:00 p.m., and 6:00 p.m. I eat two of my meals at home and one meal while I'm at work."

This will now give you specific times and places for which you'll eat at. Now you won't have to think about it every day because it's already been decided ahead of time for you.

The cool thing is that you can even take this one step farther by meal prepping. Don't worry, I cover how to go about doing this more in the chapter dedicated to meal prepping, but it really can be the difference between success and failure.

And it all comes back down to decision fatigue. Imagine this scenario, which will be happening more often than not.

You come home from work and want to eat a ketogenic meal. Then you realize that you don't have the groceries you need in order to make that meal.

In order to make this meal, you'd have to go to the store, buy the groceries, cook the meal, eat it, and clean up any dirty dishes afterwards. That's going to sound very overwhelming considering the fact that you just got home from work.

Instead, it'd be much easier to go and grab some fast food. All you have to do is drive through and pick up the food, eat it once you get home, and you're good to go.

There's nothing to clean up afterwards. In this situation, it could take more willpower to decide to make a healthy ketogenic meal than it could to actually make the meal. And like I mentioned, this is something you're going to be dealing with on most days.

It can make it hard to be successful for the long haul if you're not properly planning ahead. With meal prepping ahead of time, you can save yourself from constantly having to think about what you're going to eat, and then going through all of the effort to make the meal.

Consider the fact that if you eat three meals a day, then that means you're going to decide 3 times a day what it is you're going to eat if you take it meal-by-meal. This means you're making 21 independent decisions on what to eat throughout the week.

If you meal prep, you can cut that down considerably. You can decide on one day what all of your 21 meals will be for the week.

Now you're batching that to one day or two days, depending on how you want to meal prep. For example, imagine that on Sunday you plan ahead and prepare all of your meals for the week.

You would plan out all of the meals that you're going to eat. Then you would go to the grocery store and buy those groceries.

You would come home and batch cook for all of the meals. Now when Wednesday night rolls around and you're tired, you don't have to think.

The decision has already been made for you ahead of time when you weren't fatigued. All you have to do is take out the meal that you're going to eat, heat it up in the microwave, and you'll be good to go.

This seriously is my favorite tip to help increase your chances of success on the ketogenic diet. As far as implementation intention is concerned, you could write down the following sentence, "I meal prep all of my meals for the upcoming week on Sunday's starting at 2:00 p.m."

And don't worry, you can write down more than one sentence using the implementation intention technique. In this case, you'd be writing down how many meals you're going to eat per day, and what time you're going to eat them at.

You'd also be writing down when you're going to be preparing those meals to drastically increase your chances of success. Not only that, but if you want to add in exercise, then you could use implementation intention for that as well.

You could write down something along the lines of, "I do a 30-minute cardio workout on Monday, Wednesday, and Friday at 5:00 p.m." Essentially, any new habit that you're trying to form can benefit from using this technique of implementation intention..

And you're not limited to using it solely for your health and fitness goals. Use it for other areas of your life such as relationship and financial goals.

For example, you could say something like, "I review my financial statement once per week every Sunday at 7:00 p.m." Or for your relationship, you could say, "I take my spouse out on a date every Saturday starting at 6:00 p.m."

Finally, I want to give you a few more tips to ensure that you maximize the potential of implementation intention. Firstly, I recommend that you write it down using pen and paper.

Don't just think about it in your head or even type it. When you physically write something down it, makes it far more real than just another idea in your head that you'll eventually get around to.

You're much more engaged in the process when you write down what it is that you intend to do. The next thing you'll notice is that we're writing these sentences down in the present tense.

This helps to create a greater sense of urgency; if you say "I *will* do. . . " then it makes it easier to keep delaying the thing you know you should do. Finally, don't just write it down once and forget about it.

This technique becomes more powerful the more you write down your processes. For optimal results, write down all of the processes you're going to do morning and night.

This way it'll be the first thing on your mind and the last thing on your mind before you go to bed at night. Also, be sure to keep a copy of your implementation intention sentences at a place where you'll regularly see them.

For example, this could mean keeping a copy of them by your desk at work. This way they'll always be on the front of your mind and thus increase the chances of you following through.

The Importance of Self-Image

The next thing I want to talk about is self-image and its importance in regards to your success on the dirty ketogenic diet. Self-image is basically the way you view and think about yourself in regards to different things.

A lot of these beliefs are deep in our subconscious mind, and it affects our daily decisions. Let's use the example of money. Many of us grow up with the belief that money is hard to come by.

We're told that money doesn't grow on trees, and we act as if money is a scarce resource. If that's what we believe about money, then how hard do you think money will be to come by?

The decisions we make and how we spend it will be affected by our viewpoints on money. Another example might be someone who is shy. Maybe when growing up, this person was told by his parents and schoolteachers that he was a shy child.

Now that this person is an adult, he doesn't go out much or meet new people because he labels himself as in introvert. As long as he holds that image of being an introvert, he won't go out and meet new people for example.

He must change the way he views himself in order break out of his shyness. Finally consider two different people, each with a scar on his face.

The first person could be a war hero who sees his wound as a battle scar and is proud of the scar because it represents what he's been through. The other person might be a salesman who got into a car accident, and now his confidence is ruined because this scar is not in congruence with how he views himself.

He views himself as a handsome, well put together man. He thinks the scar makes him look less handsome; therefore, his confidence is shaken. The way he views his scar will now affect him in how he makes sales.

The subconscious mind is very powerful. It doesn't understand the difference between something that's actually happening versus something that's being vividly imagined or perceived.

Think about what we do when we worry about something. We think about something negative happening in the future and our minds think that thing is really happening or about to happen.

And if we worry enough about something, it ends up actually happening most of the time.

Our brain is like a supercomputer. It'll act on the information that we give it. Therefore, we can also feed our mind positive thoughts and outcomes, and our mind will perceive it as being real just like it does when we worry.

If we're going to think about the future, we might as well think about it in a more positive way. Using the example from earlier, the "shy person" could imagine himself having a fun and meaningful conversation with someone he just met.

However, chances are good that he probably doesn't think of having conversations with strangers in this way. He'll probably imagine himself being awkward, or not knowing what to say next; therefore, that may very be what ends up happening.

So how does all of this relate to fitness? Well, if your self-image is that of being overweight, then it doesn't matter what you do to lose weight.

Ultimately, you'll find a way to sabotage yourself and gain all of the weight back. It might seem random, but eventually you'll go back to the old self-image you have of yourself as being an overweight person.

Therefore, if the self-image doesn't change, then neither will your results. Regardless of how good this dirty keto diet plan is, you must change your self-image to that of the person you want to be.

You might not think that developing your self –image is important, and that we should focus purely on the diet itself instead. That would be a mistake because dieting isn't a purely mechanical process.

It's not as simple as me telling you what to do and then you going out and doing it. Ultimately, if you don't have the right mindset and self-image, then you won't be successful regardless of what your nutrition plan is. Now let's get into how you can actually go about changing your self-image.

How to Change Your Self-Image

In order to be able to change your self-image, you must first be able to understand what forms it in the first place. Your self-image is shaped by your past experiences.

Using our previous example of the shy person, maybe when he was a kid his parents introduced him as being shy. Unfortunately, his parents likely had no idea that they were ingraining this belief into their child.

Or maybe this person had a bad experience and was humiliated by an adult when he tried to speak up about something. That experience taught him that it's better to keep quiet rather than to speak up and be made a fool of.

Now because of these experiences, he labels himself as a shy person. That's just who he is. However, is that really true?

Will his past shyness mean that he'll always be shy for the rest of his life and that he'll never be able to become more social? Of course not!

That's why the first step that you must take when it comes to changing your self-image is to question the belief in the first place. As a matter of fact, when circuses are training elephants, they'll tether one of the elephant's feet to a pole.

When they first do this, the elephant is young and unable to break free from the rope. What's interesting is that, as time goes on, they'll use the same measly rope to tether a giant, fully grown elephant.

The elephant won't even try to break free. It's obvious to anyone who sees the elephant that it could easily break free from the rope if it simply tried to do so. We must not be like an elephant in the circus; instead, we must question the validity of our beliefs.

For example, if you've struggled to maintain a healthy body weight for most of your life, does that really mean you're destined to stay that way for the remainder of your life? Of course it doesn't.

I'm sure you might consciously know that right now as you read this; however, that's not what matters most. What matters most are the beliefs that are deeply held in your subconscious mind.

Until we can root out those myths that were planted in your subconscious mind, nothing will change. Most people know that they need to diet and exercise in order to lose weight, and yet most people aren't successful when it comes to dieting.

And the reason for that is because most people have a poor self-image. They don't believe that they're worthy of getting in shape.

And the first thing you need to do to make yourself feel worthy is to *act* worthily. Think about how you would act if you were already at your goal bodyweight.

What would your posture look like? What thoughts would you think? Would you give yourself positive or negative self-talk?

You must start to act and think as if you're already at your goal bodyweight. Right now you might be thinking, "Thomas, this sounds great and all, but it's hard for me to think of myself in a positive way when I know it's not true. It makes me feel like I'm a fraud."

In response to that, I would say it's okay if you feel that way. What you need to do is attach something you already believe about yourself to your new thoughts.

For example, let's say you're really good at planning and organizing. This skill would greatly help you out because you'll be able to meal prep on this diet.

You could then tell yourself, "I'm fit and healthy because of my ability to plan out my meals ahead of time." This is much more powerful than simply saying, "I'm fit and healthy." and having your subconscious mind balk at the idea of that.

Another example could be that you're a morning person. You might be the type of person who wakes up early seven days a week just because you like to.

If that's the case then great, you can wake up early and prepare a healthy meal or exercise with the time you have instead of waking up and feeling rushed. You could tell yourself something like, "I'm at a healthy body weight because I'm a morning person."

You might have to dig deeper than others to find something, but don't skip on this exercise. It doesn't have to be some grand thing. You could say that you're diligent, always on time, meticulous when it comes to small details, or some other positive habit, and relate that back to your new self-image. This will make the exercise much more powerful and believable to your subconscious mind.

The second thing you must do to rewire your subconscious mind is to use visualization. Remember what I said earlier—your subconscious mind doesn't know the difference between something that's actually happening versus something that's being vividly imagined.

Therefore, by using visualization you can make your subconscious mind think that this is really the way things are. And you don't have to practice this for very long.

Even just a few minutes a day will give you great benefits. For example, you could visualize yourself being at your goal bodyweight for two minutes when you wake up and another two minutes before you go to bed.

You could even do five minutes in the morning and five minutes in the evening if you want. The main point is to be consistent with it.

When you do your visualization, get really vivid with it. Make your visualizations really detailed. Involve all of your senses.

This will make the exercise much more effective. For example, what foods are you eating? What do they smell like? What do they taste like? What are your energy levels like throughout the day? What do you think you'll feel like when you're at your goal bodyweight?

Imagine yourself talking to your friends and family and them giving you compliments. Picture exactly what you'll look like and what clothes you'll wear.

You want to get as detailed with this as you possibly can. Now, it's important to mention that you must be patient with this. When you first start, your mind will tend to wander a lot.

Don't beat yourself up when you notice this happening. Instead, gently guide your mind back to the main focus, which is the visualization.

As time goes on, you'll get better and better at it, so keep at it. Thirdly, you need to shift the focus. Through these exercises, you're starting to develop a new identity of who you are.

You're starting to develop a better version of yourself. However, this doesn't mean that there won't be bumps along the way. You'll still make mistakes.

The important thing is to be careful not to let the mistakes trip you up when they do happen. When you make a mistake or do something that's incongruent with your new self, your mind won't hesitate to let you know about it.

Thoughts such as, "I knew I wasn't cut out for this", or "I knew this wouldn't last for long" are undoubtedly going to pop into your mind. Don't worry if this happens to you because it's completely normal.

Your mind is still being resistant to the idea of this new version of yourself. You must catch yourself when you notice that you're thinking these negative thoughts.

Awareness is the key here. Most people aren't even aware of what they're thinking and how it affects them. You must be different.

You must start becoming more aware of your thoughts. You'll start to notice patterns of things that upset you and start a downward spiral.

What you can do to stop a negative thought pattern? is Anchor an image of something in your head that symbolizes you needing to halt. For example, when you catch yourself thinking negative thoughts, think of something such as a big red stop sign.

This will signal you to stop thinking those thoughts. Over time, this will get more ingrained in you, and you'll get better and better at it as time goes on.

Once the negative thoughts have stopped, the next thing that you need to do is replace those negative thoughts with some positive ones. For example, you can think of some things that you've done right during the week.

Maybe on Sunday you did a good job of planning and preparing your meals for the week. When Monday comes around, you can think about how you followed through and ate everything according to the plan.

Finally, the last thing you can do to help improve your self-image is to write down your visualizations. When you're visualizing how you want to look and feel after successfully going on this dirty keto diet, write every detail of the visualization.

Writing it down will help to make things even more real for your subconscious mind. Once you're done writing it down, be sure to look at it regularly.

Really feel everything that you wrote down as you read over it. Look for similarities that are in the visualization and compare them to how you're actually living your life.

Also look for incongruencies between what you wrote down and how you're living. Use these differences to help you improve.

Improving your self-image may seem tedious and unnecessary. However, the rest of the information in this book about the dirty ketogenic diet is meaningless if you don't feel that you're worthy of being fit and achieving success.

Therefore, don't gloss over the exercises in this chapter; take them to heart and really practice them. Following through with these exercises could really make a difference in whether or not you find success on this diet.

Are you enjoying this book so far? If so, please consider leaving a review. Even just a few words would help others decide if the book is right for them.

Chapter 4: How to Overcome the Keto Flu

One thing that people commonly experience on the ketogenic diet is something known as the keto flu. Common symptoms of the keto flu include things such as fatigue, weakness, body aches, headaches, food cravings, and brain fog, among others.

The keto flu will usually occur within the first few days of you starting the diet, and it can last for days or even weeks in some cases. You might think that the keto flu is a necessary evil that you have to put up with, but as it turns out, that may not be the case...

What Causes the Keto Flu?

It's important to understand what exactly causes the keto flu to begin with. You have to remember that we're trying to make our bodies become 'fat adapted,' meaning our bodies use fat for fuel instead of carbs.

With the ketogenic diet, we want our bodies to get the energy it needs from ketone bodies, not from glucose. In order to achieve that, you must lower your carbohydrate intake and increase your fat intake.

As your body starts to lose glucose, it's also going to lose a lot of water. For every gram of carbohydrate that is stored in your body, your body will also store 2-3 grams of water along with it.

This means that when you start shedding those stored carbs, you're also going to be shedding even more water along with it. And since you're losing water, this means that you're going to be losing a lot of key electrolytes such as sodium, magnesium, and potassium.

Having a lowered amount of electrolytes in the body is what causes the keto flu to occur. Therefore, the keto flu isn't something you just have to put up with as your body starts to become fat adapted.

Instead, you can actually prevent it from occurring in the first place with the proper game plan. You'll now know ahead of time that your body is going to start losing a lot of these key electrolytes, so you can beat the keto flu to the punch by taking measures to replace the electrolytes that you're going to lose.

Even if you're not able to completely prevent these keto flu symptoms from happening, you'll know what to do if they start to occur. Obviously, I recommend that you start eating the necessary foods or taking a supplement right out of the gate when you start the ketogenic diet.

This will give you the best chance at preventing the keto flu from happening in the first place. However, if some symptoms do start to come up, then the following will help you know exactly which electrolyte could be the problem.

Sodium

This one might be hard for people to wrap their heads around because sodium generally has a bad reputation. Consuming too much sodium can be a bad thing.

Excess sodium can lead to an increase in blood pressure because you'll be holding onto excessive amounts of water. And increased blood pressure can lead to a heart attack or stroke.

On the typical American diet, people are consuming an excessive amount of sodium due to poor food choices. Not only that, but these poor food choices also contain a lot of carbs, which will make it easier for the body to retain sodium.

While too much sodium can be harmful, it also has some important functions in the body. You wouldn't want to completely get rid of it—that would be very bad!

For example, sodium helps regulate blood pressure levels. If you've ever stood up and felt light-headed, it could be because you have a low amount of sodium in your body.

Sodium is also necessary for nerve and muscle function as well as helping the body regulate the amount of water found in and around the cells. So what should you be on the lookout for to see if your body is losing too much sodium once you cut carbs?

Common symptoms of low sodium include lightheadedness upon standing up, nausea, dizziness, or muscle cramps.

So what can you do to increase your sodium intake? The first thing you might be thinking of right now is table salt, which would certainly be an easy way to increase your sodium intake.

However, I want to caution you as to what kind of salt you decide to use. Yes, this is a dirty ketogenic diet, meaning you can consume things like regular table salt and be just fine.

Even with that being the case, I want to make a plea for you to consider using something such as pink Himalayan salt or Celtic sea salt. Regular table salt is purified using a manufacturing process that heats the salt at 1,200 degrees Fahrenheit.

This process leaves you with roughly 97.5% sodium chloride and 2.5% of additives. These additives include various things such as caking agents to help prevent the salt from sticking together.

It's not just about avoiding table salt because of the additives; aside from providing you with sodium, table salt will not do anything else for you. On the other hand, pink Himalayan salt contains sodium chloride as well as 84 different minerals.

It's also natural, and it's thought to have been formed millions of years ago. Two of these minerals include potassium and magnesium, which will help you fight the keto flu.

Not only that, but pink Himalayan salt will help your body better regulate your sleep cycles and blood sugar levels. Don't get me wrong, you can certainly use regular salt on your meals if you prefer the taste of it over other types of salt.

It'll also be more convenient since you likely already have standard table salt at home. However, if you're going to go out of your way and drink salt water to increase your sodium intake, then you might as well use something like pink Himalayan salt or Celtic sea salt.

It'll provide you with more health benefits than something like regular table salt. Of course, salt isn't the only way that you can increase your sodium intake on the dirty keto diet.

You can also use something such as bone broth. Bone broth is essentially bones and connective tissue from animals that's been boiled into a broth and cooked just below boiling point for 10-20 hours.

The broth is also cooked with other things such as herbs and vegetables. Not too long ago, bone broth was something that most people consumed on a daily basis.

Nowadays, most people don't consume bone broth. It has some amazing benefits such as improving skin elasticity and skin moisture, which will help you look younger.

It'll also help with your joint health thanks to the collagen that bone broth contains. It can also help improve your gut health, among many other things.

Potassium

The next electrolyte you're going to want to make sure you get an adequate amount of is potassium. Potassium helps to regulate heart and muscle contractions, and it can also help regulate your blood pressure.

If you have a low amount of potassium, this could be why you experience things such as muscle cramps, muscle twitches, or heart palpitations. When it comes to increasing your potassium intake, what's the first thing most people think of?

Probably a banana right? Well, a banana is high in carbs and that's definitely not something that we're going to want to consume on a dirty keto diet or otherwise.

Therefore, we're going to have to get our potassium from somewhere else; don't worry, we still have some good options. Bananas aren't the only thing that are high in potassium!

As it turns out, avocados are quite high in potassium. In fact, avocados contain around 416 mg of potassium per 3 ounces. Not only that, but avocados are also a good source of healthy fats; they contain a high amount of monounsaturated fat among others.

Since this is a ketogenic diet after all, avocados really are going to be your best friend when you first start out. You'll be able to simultaneously increase your fat intake and your potassium intake by eating one food.

Of course, you're not limited to eating avocados. Greens such as spinach and kale also contain a high amount of potassium.

They contain slightly less potassium per 3 ounces than avocados, but they are still a great source nonetheless. Salmon is another food that can increase your potassium intake, although it does contain the least amount of potassium per 3 ounces at 355 mg.

That's still a good amount though, and salmon will also provide you with a good dose of Omega 3 fatty acids. This will help you improve your ratio of Omega 3's to Omega 6's, which is important since Omega 3 fatty acids act as an anti-inflammatory in the body.

Magnesium

The last electrolyte you're going to want to get an adequate amount of is magnesium. Magnesium has a lot of functions in the body, some of which include preserving muscle and nerve function, supporting the immune system, and maintaining strong bones.

Magnesium is very important for bone health, which most people don't realize. Instead, most people think of calcium when they think of keeping their bones healthy.

Yes, calcium is important for bone health, but calcium can't do its job if proper amounts of magnesium aren't present. Common symptoms you'll want to look out for to see if you have low magnesium are fatigue and muscle weakness, constipation, and an irregular heartbeat.

As far as increasing your magnesium intake is concerned, you have some good options here. The first thing you can do is supplement directly with a magnesium pill. That's an easy way to increase your magnesium intake without having to put any thought into what foods you're eating.

If you want to increase your magnesium intake through your diet, then you still have plenty of keto-friendly options. Various seeds like flax or pumpkin seeds are high in magnesium.

Different kinds of nuts such as almonds are also high in magnesium. Finally, foods such as spinach, mackerel, salmon, and avocados are also high in magnesium.

And as you'll recall, some of these foods (spinach, salmon, and avocados) are also high in potassium, so you can get the most bang for your buck by eating those kinds of foods.

Lastly, you can also supplement directly with electrolytes. Typically, you'll get this in a powder form that you can mix with some water, and you'll be good to go.

Of course, you don't have to supplement with electrolytes if you don't want to. You can easily meet all of your electrolyte needs from dietary food sources alone if you prefer.

Chapter 5: How to Eat Keto at Restaurants, Parties, or Other Social Events

When people start a ketogenic diet, things go well for the first couple of weeks. Then life happens and some sort of event will come up.

Maybe your work decides to cater lunch, you have a wedding to attend, or some other social event is coming up. You tell yourself that you've been following the diet very well for the past couple of weeks, so what could one cheat meal hurt?

You'll get right back on track tomorrow and be back in ketosis before you know it. Next thing you know, tomorrow turns into a week, which turns into a month, and you still haven't gone back to eating keto.

Like I talked about in a previous chapter, it can be hard to get back into keto once you've lost momentum. Don't worry though, in this chapter I'm going to give you some helpful tips and tricks to help you stay on track with your dirty ketogenic diet when you're put in tough situations.

This is the Number One Key for Success on the Dirty Keto Diet

The best thing you can do to ensure success on the dirty keto diet is plan, plan, plan. Being prepared for the given situation is your best line of defense against slipping up on this diet.

What tends to happen on the ketogenic diet is that people get caught in tough, unexpected situations. It can be something like a co-worker bringing cookies to work, or it could something as simple as you being too tired to cook after a long day at work.

These are the types of things that you have to think about in advance. For example, if you know you're going to be too tired to cook after work, then you need to meal prep in advance.

This is critical. It's why I've dedicated an entire chapter to meal prepping; it can make or break your success. In the case of a co-worker bringing cookies to work, you have to remember that you can't eat anything that's high in sugar on this diet plan.

Therefore, if this is something that happens regularly, you need to put a rule into place that says you're not allowed to eat anything high in carbs that your coworkers bring to work.

If that's not good enough and you still find yourself being tempted by peer pressure or something else, then take things one-step further. Set a hard rule in place that states you're not allowed to eat anything your coworkers bring to work. Period.

You only eat the food that you bring to work. This way the decision is made for you in advance, and you don't have to think or worry about it. The same principle of planning in advance will apply to whatever situation you find yourself in.

Sometimes things will come up suddenly, and you'll need to be able to adapt to the given situation. In these instances, you'll have to do your best with what you've got.

However, there are a lot of situations that you'll know are happening in advance. For example, there might be an upcoming party this weekend.

When you find yourself in these types of situations, you must do your best to prepare in advance for what's to come. Here are some helpful tips you can follow that will help you out in various situations you may find yourself in.

What to Do at Parties or Other Social Events

Let's say there's a work Christmas party or some other social event that you know of in advance. What can you do to make sure that you follow your dirty keto diet in these situations?

The first thing you need to do is get in contact with the host. Ask him or her what kinds of food will be at the party. If there are low-carb keto type of foods available, then you know you'll be okay.

If not, then ask if there can be any accommodations made for a low-carb high fat diet that you're currently on. Even if the host isn't able to help you out, there are still a couple of things you can do.

The first would be to ask if it's okay if you bring your own dish to the party. You could explain how you're not the only person at the party who's on a keto diet so other people will enjoy the dish as well.

If that's not an option, there's one of two things you can still do. The first would be to eat a keto meal before you go to the party.

This way you won't be hungry, and you'll be far less tempted to eat something that you shouldn't. The other option you have would be to prepare a keto meal in advance and eat it at the party.

The idea of doing this certainly sounds intimidating. However, if you simply explain to anyone who asks what it is that you're doing, they should be understanding.

Just explain how you're on a keto diet, which is a low-carb and high-fat diet. This is what allows your body to get into ketosis, which is where your body uses fat for fuel instead of carbs.

If you explain this with enthusiasm and passion, you could very well convince other people at the event to start a ketogenic diet! You have to have confidence in what you're doing.

In all actuality, most people won't care what it is that you're eating, or even notice in the first place. If you want proof of this, simply ask yourself if you remember what everyone else ate, drank, and wore to a party that you've been to before.

Chances are good you barely remember any of that stuff! You were probably far more concerned with what *you* were going to eat, drink, and wear to the party.

Once again, you may notice that sticking to your diet plan at parties comes down to planning in advance.

While it may be easier to simply show up to the party and hope that there's something keto approved that you could eat, take the time to plan ahead. Instead of being a victim to the circumstances, you can take matters into your own hands and ensure that you'll be able to stick to your diet plan.

How to Eat Keto at Fast Food Restaurants

Up next we have the common fast food restaurant. Depending on what restaurant you're eating at will determine your game plan, so I want to cover as many different kinds as I can in this section.

The first tip would be to look and see if the place you're eating at has salads on the menu. This can be a great way to consume more greens and eat keto when you're on the go.

However, you have to be careful because not all salads are the same. The main culprit here you need to watch out for is the salad dressing.

Any type of sweet salad dressing such as a raspberry or balsamic vinaigrette will be too high in sugar for you to eat. Ideally, you'll want to add olive oil to the salad that you're eating.

However, any other high-fat dressing such as blue cheese and Caesar dressing would also be acceptable.

Next up are restaurants that serve pizza. This one is tricky because of the crust that contains a lot of carbs. Your best choice would be to eat a cauliflower crust pizza.

This will allow you to eat pizza while avoiding the carbs. However, most pizza places won't serve cauliflower pizza unless it's a specialty restaurant.

Therefore, we're most likely going to have to get creative. The first thing you want to do is load up the pizza with as many keto-approved toppings as possible.

This way you'll be able to fill yourself up on the toppings and not be as tempted to eat something you shouldn't. Next, you want to eat the cheese and toppings on the pizza while avoiding the crust.

This can be hard to do; the best way to go about it would be to use a fork or knife to separate the cheese and toppings from the crust. Finally, you might be able to order thin crust and get away with it depending on how much pizza you plan on eating.

If you're going to do this, make sure that you check the nutrition info first. If the crust contains too many carbs, then you're going to have to pass on it.

In this case, it would simply be better to order a hand tossed pizza. It'll be much easier to separate the cheese and toppings from a hand tossed pizza compared to a thin crust pizza.

Overall though, trying to eat pizza on a ketogenic diet isn't the best idea or the easiest thing to do. If it's possible to eat somewhere else, then you should definitely do that.

However, if you do find yourself at a pizza restaurant, this is the best way to survive while you're following a ketogenic diet.

Up next we have restaurants that serve burgers. This is probably one of the more popular food items you'll see at restaurants in America.

So how can you eat keto at a burger restaurant? The best way to go about things is to order a lettuce wrap.

This is starting to become more and more popular even though a lot of restaurants have yet to catch on. Essentially, the burger is wrapped in lettuce, which is used in place of a bun.

This will help save you on the calories and carbs and allow you to stay in ketosis. As I mentioned before, not all burger places have lettuce wraps, so what should you do in these cases?

Well, the best way to go about things would be to simply pull the bun back slightly and eat the burger in little bites while avoiding the bun. This way you still get the feel of eating a regular burger and the bun will still be able to hold everything in place.

You could also grab a fork and knife and cut up the meat in small pieces and eat that with the toppings in a similar manner to a salad. Now as far as sides are concerned, you're definitely going to have to pass on the fries and soda.

If the restaurant sells a lettuce wrap, then there's a chance that they might have some better side options you can replace the fries with. You might be able to get a side of steamed broccoli or kale chips with your burger instead of fries.

Worst case scenario though, you might not be able to get any sides at all. Even with that being the case, at least it's still possible to eat keto at a burger restaurant.

What about Mexican restaurants? How do you go about eating keto at a Mexican restaurant?

Well as with a lot of things so far, there are some sacrifices that you're going to have to make. However, there are also plenty of good options available to you that'll allow you to still be able to maintain your dirty ketogenic diet.

The first thing that you're going to have to do no matter how difficult is avoid the tortilla chips that are served before your meal. Even if you're eating them with something that contains a low amount of carbs such as guacamole, the chips aren't keto approved; if you eat too many of them, you'll run the risk of getting kicked out of ketosis.

Don't worry, things get much better from here. The first thing you can do is see if you can order your food in a bowl. This is essentially where they take all of the ingredients that they'd normally wrap in a burrito (such as the meat, vegetables, and keto approved sauces that you're adding) and put it into a bowl instead.

This is great because it's very similar to what you'd be doing at a burger restaurant except in this case, it'll be much easier to eat. Even if the place you're eating at doesn't offer a bowl option, then you can simply order a burrito with everything you want inside of it.

Then when you get your food, you can unwrap the burrito and eat the contents with a fork. You can do the same thing with fajitas. Simply order the fajitas, but when the food arrives, don't use any of the tortillas that come with the meal.

If you're eating at a place that predominantly sells tacos, you can still do the same thing. You can remove the contents of the taco from the shell and eat them with a fork, almost like you would with a salad.

Your choice of sides may be more limited. Most Mexican restaurants serve rice and beans as their primary sides, and there's usually not much variation to that.

If that's the case, you're definitely going to have to skip out on those sides at the place you're eating at. Instead, see if the restaurant offers the option to double the meats with whatever it is that you're ordering.

If they don't, then your best option would be to order two main courses without the sides or do one main order and load it up with as many vegetables as possible.

Finally, we have Asian restaurants. This is the hardest place to eat at on a keto diet. Things that would normally be keto approved (such as certain meats) aren't in these places because of the way that they're typically prepared.

A lot of the time, these meats will either be breaded or lathered in a sauce that will cause them to contain too many carbs. Cornstarch is another ingredient that's commonly used when preparing Asian dishes, and it's certainly not keto approved.

Therefore, it can be easy to think you're eating keto at an Asian restaurant when in reality, you're not. Additionally, two of the main components of an Asian meal are often going to be fried rice or chow mein.

Neither of these are keto-approved, and that's going to make things a lot more difficult. Another popular side item at Asian restaurants is egg rolls, but again, these aren't keto approved either.

So what can you eat at an Asian restaurant? The first thing would be chicken and broccoli. This is something that a lot of Asian restaurants will have.

The trick is in how it's made. You need to make sure the meat isn't breaded, and you need to ask if it can be served with a keto-approved sauce on the side.

Next up you can see if the place you're eating at serves lettuce wraps. You'll have to double check to see how all of the contents are prepared inside, but it's an option if everything checks out.

And finally we have egg drop soup. Again, this all comes down to how the dish is prepared. Cornstarch is frequently used to make the soup, and it definitely won't be keto if that's the case.

When it comes to eating keto at restaurants, there are some much better options to pick over Asian food. The main reason why people like it in the first place is because of the rice, chow mein, and sauces that are used.

You're not going to be able to eat any of these things on a ketogenic diet anyway, so it's best to avoid Asian restaurants if at all possible. At least in the case of a burger or Mexican restaurant, you're still able to eat the main contents of the meal without any worries about how it was prepared most of the time.

In the case of the Asian restaurant, it's the exact opposite. The dishes will usually be made in a way that doesn't make the food keto-approved anymore.

It's simply best to avoid the temptation altogether in the first place. Once you're in a restaurant and you're ready to order, it can be very hard to leave at that point if they're not going to be able to accommodate to your needs.

This makes it all the more likely that you're going to cheat on your diet plan. You're better off avoiding a sticky situation in the first place if you can help it.

Hopefully these tips gave you some good ideas for how you can eat keto when you're eating at restaurants. Remember, the main thing you want to focus on is being prepared.

That's going to be your best line of defense against eating something that isn't keto approved. Even with that being the case, there will still be times when you're on the go and have to do the best you can with what you've got. That's where these tips will really shine, so be sure to keep them in mind!

Chapter 6: The Importance of Sleep and Why It Can Make or Break Your Success

In this chapter, I'm going to go in depth about why sleep is so important for your fat loss success. You might not think that this is necessary, but it definitely is.

Think about it—you're going to follow this dirty ketogenic diet for a reason right? What is that reason? Are you doing it to feel better and have more energy?

Are you following this keto plan so that you can lose weight? To improve your health? Whatever the reason is, I can assure you that what you eat isn't the only thing that affects your energy levels or your weight.

I don't want this book to be something that simply tells you about the dirty keto diet and then leaves you hoping for the best. I know that there's a certain outcome you want to obtain.

I also know that without a proper mindset or good sleeping habits, you will still fail, even if you follow a great nutrition plan.

In fact, the quantity and quality of your sleep could affect your success more than your diet does. If you're not getting an adequate amount of sleep on a regular basis, then you're going to be fighting an uphill battle in regards to losing weight.

This is because sleep affects key hormones that regulate hunger and how much fat you burn. For this reason, sleep is something you want to take very seriously.

In fact, I'd say sleep is the most important aspect of maintaining a healthy body, followed by your diet, and then exercise. The reason for this is because you're going to spend approximately one-third of your life sleeping.

You'll spend far less time eating and exercising. Therefore, it makes sense to get your sleeping habits in check.

However, most people struggle to get enough sleep at night. We're constantly on the move, always too busy or too stressed out to get a good night's rest; even though it's so important, sleep always seems to take the biggest hit.

We try to make up for the lack of sleep with caffeine, but that can often make things worse depending on when its taken. Before I get into what you need to start doing in order to improve the quality and quantity of your sleep, let's first talk about why sleep is so important to begin with.

Why Sleep Greatly Matters if You Want to Burn Fat

So how much sleep should you be getting on a nightly basis? The research consistently shows that adults need to get around 7-9 hours of sleep per night for optimal health (3).

Even with this being the case, there are still are a lot of people out there who are only getting 6 or even 5 hours of sleep per night. This shouldn't come as a surprise though, as we are busier now more than ever before.

With all of the hustle and bustle that goes on in today's world, something will most likely have to be sacrificed. Hopefully I can make a compelling case for you to prioritize sleep over other things if you're serious about achieving your health and fitness goals.

Firstly, let's focus on how sleep affects your body's ability to burn fat. The first hormones I want to start with are cortisol and melatonin.

You can think of these hormones as opposites in a way. Cortisol signals stress to the body.

If you think about being in fight-or-flight mode, it would be because your body is secreting a high amount of cortisol. When you think of cortisol, you might think of stress and negative things, but cortisol isn't all bad.

The body wouldn't produce something that's purely harmful to itself all of the time. Cortisol is responsible for regulating your body's sleep/wake cycle, your blood sugar levels, and your metabolism.

Cortisol also helps to reduce inflammation. Cortisol creates issues when you produce too much of it at the wrong time, or too much of it too often.

Excessive cortisol levels can cause fatigue, headaches, anxiety, and weight gain, among other things. Ideally, cortisol levels will be at their highest in the morning when you need to wake up and get going for the day.

They should be the lowest when you're trying to go to bed. Melatonin, as I mentioned earlier, can be seen as an opposite to cortisol.

Melatonin helps to regulate sleep/wake cycles by signaling to the body when to relax and rest. Think of melatonin as putting your body in a restful parasympathetic state, whereas cortisol will put your body into a heightened fight-or-flight sympathetic state.

Because of this, it's most ideal to have your melatonin levels be at their highest at night after the sun goes down, and at their lowest in the morning when you're trying to wake up.

Of course, melatonin is responsible for other things, but our primary concern here is how melatonin regulates our sleep cycles. Back in the old days, we would sleep in accordance with the sun.

When the sun rose, we would wake up. When the sun would set, we would go to sleep. This internal and natural cycle that regulates sleepiness and alertness is known as your circadian rhythm or biological clock.

There weren't very many things people could do productivity wise once the sun went down. Nowadays with modern technology, things are much different.

We have artificial light sources that we can use to still get things done during all hours of the day. This might be great for productivity purposes, but it's thrown our hormones and our biological clocks out of whack.

This means that our sleep quality has suffered in recent times. Therefore, the first thing you need to do to improve your sleep quality is to get your biological clock back on track.

The easiest way to do that is to rise with the sun and sleep when the sun sets. Of course, depending on where you live and how much sunlight you get per day, this might not be practical.

The next best thing you could do is sleep during times that are more in accordance with your circadian rhythm. For example, you could go to bed at 10:00 p.m. and wake up at 6:00 a.m.

Or maybe sleeping around 11:00 p.m and waking around 7:00 a.m better fits your schedule. The point is to get to bed earlier and wake up earlier.

Have you ever gone to bed at 2:00 a.m. and woken up at 10:00 a.m. still feeling super tired even though you got eight hours of sleep? I know that I sure have before, but now it makes sense why this happens.

Going to bed at 2:00 a.m. and waking up at 10:00 a.m. completely throws your biological clock out of whack. It causes your body to produce more cortisol at night and less melatonin.

Then you'll be sleeping and your body will be producing less cortisol than it needs to when it's time to wake up. Typically when we stay up late, we're not doing anything productive anyway.

More than likely we're either watching television, or we are on our phones. These electronic devices emit something known as blue light.

Blue light is shorter in wavelength, which causes it to produce more energy. The sun is a producer of blue light, but even after the sun has gone down we can still get exposure to artificial blue light, all thanks to our electronic devices like televisions, cell phones, tablets, and game systems.

The problem with staying on these devices late at night is the fact that blue light exposure will suppress melatonin production because this light spectrum will stimulate alertness. This will not only affect the quality of your sleep, but it will also make it harder for you to fall asleep in the first place.

So what can you do to stop exposure to blue light late at night? The first option you have is to buy some blue light blocking glasses.

These glasses have an orange tint to them, which will help to block the blue light wavelength. Yes, it'll make everything else have a weird coloration to it, but it's worth it if it'll help improve the quality of your sleep.

The cool thing about the glasses is that you can put them on and not have to worry about anything. It doesn't matter if you watch t.v., get on your phone, or play video games—you'll be covered.

Ideally, you'd start to wear these glasses three hours before you go to bed. So if you were going to go to bed at 10:30 p.m., you'd start to wear the glasses at 7:30 p.m.

If the glasses aren't your style, then that's completely fine. Most devices will allow you to download a blue light blocking filter.

For example, you can download an app on your smart phone that will block the blue light that's emitted from your phone. It'll give your phone screen more of an orange tint to it, but it's worth putting up with for the better quality sleep.

The cool thing is that you can set the filter to come on and off at certain times so you don't even have to think about it. The same can also be said for your computer.

You can download a software and have it set to come on at a certain time to block the blue light that's emitted from it. One downside to this is that you may not be able to do this for all of your devices.

Most televisions and video games systems don't have a way for you to be able to block the blue light that comes from them. Sure, you may be covered on some devices such as your smartphone, but if you decide to watch t.v., then you'll still be getting blue light exposure late at night.

That's why I think the glasses are the best way to go. They might not be the most fashionable thing, but most of the time you'll be wearing them late in the day in the comfort of your own home.

You can wear them and forget about the rest regardless of what you're doing. The thing is that blue light can sneak up on us in a lot of different ways that we might not realize.

For instance, the lights you use in your home could stimulate you to stay awake. The glow from your computer or alarm clock could be another culprit.

Or maybe you could look at something on someone else's electronic device and be exposed to blue light in that way. All of these things will affect your body's ability to produce melatonin at night, so you'll want to make sure you avoid blue light during the night as much as you possibly can.

Something you might be thinking of doing right now to get around this would be to take a melatonin supplement. This can be tempting, but I would completely avoid it.

The reason why people commonly take this supplement is because of poor sleep quality. However, when you're taking a melatonin supplement, all you're really doing is addressing a symptom and not the root cause.

For example, you might consistently wake up feeling tired and drowsy and not know why. So you decide to take a melatonin supplement in the hopes that it'll give you better sleep and fix the issue.

It might work for a while, but the real reason that you're waking up tired could be caused by something such as blue light exposure, or you not getting enough sleep at night. These are the real issues that need to be addressed.

You're suppressing your melatonin secretion late at night by being on electronic devices, and then you're trying to make up for it by taking a supplement. This isn't even the main reason why you shouldn't take a melatonin supplement.

The thing is that melatonin is naturally produced by the body. What do you think is going to happen once you start getting your melatonin from an outside source?

Your body will know that you already have plenty of melatonin in your system and that it doesn't need to make any more. Therefore your body will begin to stop the natural production of melatonin.

Not only that, but as times goes on, you'll need to take more and more melatonin in order to get the same effects. When you initially start taking melatonin, you won't need to supplement with that much of it because your body will still be producing high amounts of it.

Over time though, your body will start to decline the amount of melatonin that it's producing. This means that you're going to have to take more melatonin in order to make up for that difference.

Later on down the line, you more than likely won't be able to stop taking melatonin cold turkey. That would completely wreck your sleep cycle. Instead, you'd have to gradually wean yourself off of it in order to signal to your body to start producing melatonin again.

And finally, it's not as if supplements are free. It could cost you quite a bit of money over the long haul if you take a melatonin supplement.

This is why you're better off not taking it in the first place if at all possible. The only exception to this would be if you work a graveyard shift or something similar.

In this case, you're already going to be going against your body's biological clock because you'll be working when you should be naturally sleeping. In this case, taking melatonin will help to put your body in a relaxed and restful state during a time when melatonin production is usually low and cortisol production is higher.

Melatonin and cortisol aren't the only two hormones you need to worry about as far as good sleep is concerned. Not sleeping enough and poor sleep quality affect other hormones as well.

Two big ones are leptin and ghrelin. You can think of these hormones as opposites, similar to melatonin and cortisol.

Leptin is your body's satiety hormone. When leptin is high, it signals to the body that you have enough stored fat and that you don't need to eat any more food.

When leptin is low, this will signal to the body that you don't have enough stored fat and your body will try to conserve energy in an attempt to prevent you from starving to death.

This was great back in the hunter and gatherer days because our ancestors usually didn't know where their next meal was going to come from. Leptin allowed them to hold onto the stored fat that they had in case of an emergency.

In today's world, things are much different. We have food at our fingertips 24/7. We have food in our fridge that we can access anytime time we're at home.

There are plenty of grocery stores and restaurants that are open 24 hours a day. In first world countries, there is no shortage of food.

Regardless of this being the case, our hormones haven't gotten the message. Even if you have plenty of extra stored body fat and plenty of access to food, your body will still act in the same manner.

Your body will want to hold onto that stored fat in case there's a long period of time where you won't have access to food. So if your sleep is out of whack, that's also going to make your leptin levels out of whack.

You definitely don't want your body holding onto your stored fat if it can be prevented in the first place. We also have ghrelin. Like I mentioned earlier, ghrelin acts in a manner opposite to that of leptin.

Ghrelin is your body's hunger hormone. It signals to the body that you're hungry. When you're not feeling hungry, ghrelin levels will be low; when you're feeling, hungry ghrelin levels will be high.

Sleep deprivation will cause an increase in ghrelin and a decrease in leptin. This basically means that you're fighting an uphill battle with your body's hormones.

Under normal circumstances, you might not have these intense feelings of hunger. However, if you're deprived of sleep, then you could be hungry at a time when you normally wouldn't be.

In addition to that, lack of sleep will also affect your willpower. Imagine for instance that you get plenty of sleep.

You wake up feeling good about yourself, you exercise for a bit, and eat a healthy breakfast. How likely do you think it is that you're going to eat a good keto meal for lunch and dinner that day?

How likely is it that you'll be able to avoid tempting foods that your coworkers may bring to work? The answer to that is pretty darn likely.

You're feeling good about yourself, and you've been able to build momentum at the very start of your day. This is all because you got plenty of sleep at night and you're now able to make better decisions as the day goes on.

Now compare that scenario to something much different. Let's say this time you don't get a good night's sleep.

Maybe there was something really stressful at work or something came up with your family which caused you to only get 5 hours of sleep that night. What do you think is going to happen the next day?

Well, more than likely you're going to wake up feeling rushed because you'll want to sleep in for as long as possible. You hit the snooze button a few times before getting up.

Then once you did get up, you found yourself rushing to get to work on time. You didn't have any time to eat a healthy breakfast or exercise before work.

Then once you're at work, you're probably going to feel hungrier and more irritable than you usually do thanks to the increased ghrelin. Now when your coworker brings cookies for everyone to eat at lunch, you're far more likely to indulge.

You might find yourself already eating the cookie before you even realize what's going on. Then once you realize how eating this cookie goes against your diet plan, you'll start to feel guilty about yourself and tailspin out of control, possibly taking weeks before you get things back on track.

And this was all because your sleep got thrown off the night before. A lot of times when it comes to dieting, people only tend to think about the mechanical part of the process.

For example, people think about what they need to eat, what they need to avoid, and if they stick to that, they will be good to go. What people often fail to think about is how we're making the decisions that we are.

For instance, someone might think that he or she is bad at following a diet plan because of consistently failing to be able to stick to anything. The truth is that it could all be because of some other factor; Perhaps a poor self-image or lack of sleep is holding the person back from making the correct decision.

Hopefully you now see the importance of getting enough quality sleep at night. Now the question becomes what you can do to improve your sleep quality and quantity at night.

How to Improve Your Sleep Quality and Quantity at Night

Getting enough sleep is a big factor in the equation of our health and fat loss journey. Even if you're getting 4 hours of quality sleep each and every night, that won't be long enough for you to get the full benefits of sleep.

You need to make sure that you're falling into that 7-9 hour range that we talked about earlier. One of the main reasons for this is because our body sleeps in cycles.

There are 5 different stages of sleep. The first stage is a light sleep, and the second stage prepares the body for the deep sleep that comes during stages 3 and 4. The last stage is rapid eye movement sleep (REM).

During the final stage of REM sleep, the eyes are still closed, but your eyes are rapidly moving as the name implies. Each sleep cycle will typically take around 90 minutes or so.

Ideally, you'd want to wake up at the completion of a sleep cycle. For you, this could mean getting 7.5 hours of sleep per night or even 9. It really depends though, as some sleep cycles are slightly longer than 90 minutes; if that's the case, 8 hours of sleep might be right for you.

You'll have to test it out and see what works best for you. And if you've ever gotten plenty of sleep, yet you still woke up tired, then it could be because you woke up during a deep stage of sleep such as stage 3 or 4.

If you're only getting 5 hours of sleep per night for instance, then you're not giving your body much of a chance to complete the correct number of sleep cycles that it needs to. Not only is sleep important for fat loss purposes, but you also need sleep for other things.

Sleep helps your immune system function properly. It's definitely going to be harder to reach your fitness goals if you're regularly getting sick.

And sleep is also important for memory consolidation. If you're sleep deprived, then you'll have a harder time retaining information compared to someone who's getting an adequate amount of sleep each night.

Now let's talk about what you can do to increase the amount of time that you're sleeping each night if you're currently struggling with that. The first tip would be to see what time you're usually going to bed at night.

If you need to get more sleep at night, the first solution is to start going to bed earlier, although this is typically easier said than done. Usually, this is where the problem lies; you have to get up early for work, but you're going to bed too late.

See when it is that you're generally going to bed, and notice what you are doing late at night. Are you using the electronic devices that are stimulating you to stay awake?

Maybe you're eating foods late at night that are causing you to stay up. Whatever it is, you need to become aware of it so you can fix the problem.

For example, it's going to be hard to go to bed earlier if you're on your phone late at night. Therefore, the first thing that you must do is cut out distractions late at night.

You don't want to be doing anything that can stimulate you to stay up later than you're supposed to. Even if you're using blue-light blocking glasses, things such as social media on your phone can be easy to scroll through endlessly; next thing you know, it's suddenly an hour past your bedtime.

That's why you're better off following the rule of no electronic devices an hour before bedtime. This will make things much easier for you to be able to get to bed on time.

When I was trying to get a consistent sleep schedule down, I really struggled. Eventually I realized that I struggled because I kept watching videos on my phone late at night. One video would lead to the next and before I knew it, it was 2 a.m.

Even with the blue light filter on, it didn't matter. My phone was distracting me from getting to bed on time.

My solution to this problem was to set an alarm for when it was time for me to start getting ready to go to bed. Most people only set alarms for when it's time to wake up, but why not set an alarm to alert you when it's time to go to bed as well?

I go to bed around 10:30 p.m. every night, so I set an alarm for 9:30 p.m. This tells me to stop the use of all electronic devices and to start getting ready for bed.

My phone even has a feature that'll lock me out of any potentially distracting apps. After you do that, you'll definitely want to make sure that you go to bed and wake up at the same time every day of the week.

This is actually the most important tip for improving your sleep quality and energy levels. Think about what it is that most people do.

They'll wake up at the same time 5 days per week to go to work, but they will sleep in during the weekend. You're not giving your body a consistent schedule to adapt to when you do that.

Your body starts to adjust to waking up around 7:00 a.m. every day. Then the weekend comes around and you sleep in until 10:30 a.m, and suddenly your body is confused. When Monday comes around, your body will be stuck trying to wake up at 10:30 a.m instead of 7:00 a.m.

Your body won't know what to think. You'll likely wake up a little tired on Monday because you're trying to get back into the swing of things.

You probably won't get back on track until Wednesday, but by Friday night you'll throw things all out of whack again. The only solution to this is to wake up at the same time every single day of the week.

A more structured sleep will allow your body to know when it's time to start producing melatonin at night and when it's time to start producing cortisol in the morning. I know you might be turned off to the idea of this, but I promise it works.

Before I did this, I was always tired and frequently took naps. Now I wake up feeling well rested, and I feel energized throughout the day.

Of course, you might be wondering, what am I supposed to do on the weekends when I wake up early? Well, there are plenty of things to do!

You could do something relaxing such as reading a book. You could exercise, or you could start your meal prepping for the week.

The point is that you want to find something, and it needs to be important. Personally, if what I'm doing in the morning isn't that important to me, then I'm far more likely to sleep in.

I'm willing to bet that you might be the same way. If reading a book doesn't sound that appealing to you at 7:00 a.m. on a Saturday morning, then you'll need to find something else.

Meal prepping is a really solid option to do during this time. It's important, and it'll help set you up for a good week on the keto diet plan.

You'll get it out of the way first thing in the morning, and you'll have time during the rest of the day to do whatever it is that you want. You could even split up your meal prepping during Saturday and Sunday mornings so that you have something to do on both days.

If you did this, you'd set yourself up for major success on the ketogenic diet. Of course, meal prepping isn't your only option.

You just need to find something you're interested in doing during your weekend mornings. If you find yourself struggling to get started with this tip, there are a couple of things that you can do.

The first thing is to make sure that you set your alarm clock across the room from where you sleep before you go to bed. For example, if you use your phone as an alarm clock, then set it across the room so that you have to get out of your bed in order to turn it off in the morning.

This will also help prevent you from staying on your phone late at night. If it's within arms reach, then it's far too easy to turn the alarm off and go back to bed.

This is a simple tip but it works wonders. Now you might be thinking, "Thomas, I've tried that before and it didn't work!" Perhaps you would just get up, turn off my alarm, and then go right back to bed.

If this is the case, you'll need to get more creative. For example, you might need to buy a special light that can be controlled through an app on your phone. These light bulbs aren't that expensive either (usually $20 or less) and you can program the light to come on during a certain time of the day.

If you're trying to get up at 7:00 a.m., then you could set the light to come on at 7:00 a.m. and have your alarm go off at that time as well. If that's still not enough, then get multiple alarm clocks and set them up in opposite corners in your room.

Then when all of them go off at once, it'll be really loud and you'll be wide awake by the time you turn all of them off. Secondly, get excited the night before, as if you have something to really look forward to in the morning.

Think about a kid on Christmas morning. Are they thinking negative thoughts before going to bed that night? No, of course not!

They're full of energy and ready to go at 5 or 6 in the morning because they can't wait to open presents! However, as adults, we typically think about how we aren't going to get a lot of sleep after getting home late, or how tired we will be in the morning after only sleeping a few hours.

Instead of thinking thoughts about how tired we're going to be in the morning, why not think in the opposite manner?

Think about things such as, "I'm getting plenty of sleep tonight. I'm going to wake up tomorrow fully rested and full of energy!" You'll want to do this regardless of how much sleep it is that you're going to be getting that night.

While you ideally want to get 7-9 hours of sleep per night, there will still be some nights where you don't hit that number. These are the nights when thinking positive thoughts before bed will come in handy.

You can even go as far as practicing waking up excited during the middle of the day. I've done this before, and it works really well. Simply set your alarm for one minute past the current time and then when it goes off, spring out of bed with excitement.

By doing this, you're starting to train your brain to view your alarm as a positive thing, not a negative thing. If you currently view your alarm ringtone as negative, then change it to something else.

This way you can start to associate that ring with positive feelings and thoughts rather than negative ones. The main thing is to be creative and not make excuses; this tip of waking up at the same time every day can make or break your success.

Now let's get into some more specific tips you can do to improve your sleep quality at night. A lot of these tips work hand-in-hand with each other as far as sleep quality and quantity is concerned.

For example, drinking caffeine late at night will affect both your sleep quality and quantity. Caffeine is a good place to start.

You definitely don't want to consume any caffeine at least 10 hours before you go to bed. For example, if you're going to bed at 11:00 p.m., then you don't want to consume any caffeine past 1:00 p.m.

It might not sound too harmful to drink coffee later than that, but the thing most people don't realize is that caffeine stays in your system for hours after you drink it. Therefore, that coffee you had in the late afternoon could be affecting your sleep later that night.

Some people might try to mask this issue by taking melatonin, but the better thing to do would be to stop drinking coffee so late in the day. If you're drinking coffee that late to become more alert, then there's something deeper with your sleep that needs to be fixed Drinking more coffee isn't the solution.

Another thing you'll want to avoid doing is drinking alcohol late at night. This is a keto diet so most alcohol isn't keto-approved anyway, however, you do still have some options that I'll cover later on.

For now though, understand that alcohol and the quality of your sleep don't go hand-in-hand. Sure, drinking some alcohol might put your body in a relaxed state and make it easier for you to fall asleep, but you'll pay the price during the night.

Alcohol affects your REM sleep, which can cause you to wake up in the middle of the night, snore, and sleepwalk during the night. When you wake up, you might feel groggy and irritable.

Aside from avoiding alcohol and caffeine, something you can do to help you fall asleep faster is to start a journal. No, I'm not talking about keeping a journal like a teenager going through a breakup.

Instead, we're going to use this journal to help get all of our thoughts down on paper before bedtime. Whenever you try to go to sleep, have you ever noticed how your mind is racing with thoughts?

You could spend 30 minutes just thinking of different things about your day before you're able to actually fall asleep. Well, journaling at night before you go to bed will help with that.

Just do a complete brain dump of anything you're thinking about and write it down. Don't even think, just keep writing for 5 minutes straight and get everything down on the paper.

Then when it's time to go to bed, you should notice that your mind is a lot calmer and that it's much easier to fall asleep. There's something special about putting your thoughts down on paper that helps calm down our brain.

These final two tips might not seem that important, but they can make a big difference. The first one is to make sure that you're clean before you go to bed. Research shows that we sleep better at night when we're clean (4). This means that you need to take a shower at night before going to bed in order to improve your sleep quality.

I understand that a lot of people might take a shower in the morning. The shower might be used as a way to wake up and get their morning started.

However, if you think about it, it makes more sense to take a shower before bed. This way you won't go to sleep at night feeling dirty or smelly, which will help improve the quality of your sleep at night.

Not only that, but if you're taking showers in the morning as a way to help wake yourself, you'll no longer need to do that if you're following the other tips I've talked about. Finally, the last thing you need to do in order to improve your sleep quality is to make your bedroom as dark as possible when you're going to bed.

You don't want any light coming from computer screens, televisions, alarm clocks, or night lights in your room. The reason for this is because these blue lights will affect your body's ability to produce melatonin at night. This will obviously impact the quality of your sleep.

If implementing all of these tips at once sounds overwhelming to you, then only start with a few of them. Try out the ones you think will have the biggest impact on your sleep and then go from there.

For instance, you could start by placing your phone across the room when you sleep and avoiding electronic devices for at least an hour before you go to bed. After you've gotten those habits down, you can move onto something else such as waking up at the same time every day of the week.

The best thing you can do in regards to your sleep is to take action on some or all of these habits now. Don't delay. I know first hand how easy it can be to put off better sleep habits until the next night, and trust me it's not worth it.

Chapter 7: How to Meal Prep on a Ketogenic Diet

Meal prepping is the single most important thing that you can do in order to drastically increase your chances of success on the dirty ketogenic diet. The reason for this is because you failing to prepare is setting you up to fail.

Meal prepping essentially takes all of the decisions and work you'd have to do during the week and condenses it down into one or two days. A lot of this has to do with decision fatigue as I talked about in an earlier chapter.

This is something most people don't know about, and therefore it's not a threat they see coming that can ruin their success. For example, if you're eating 3 meals a day each day of the week, then that's a total of 21 meals per week.

For most people, this would mean that they're making 21 individual decisions about what they want to eat. Then they have to get the necessary ingredients to make whatever meal it is they want to eat. After that, they have to prepare the meal, eat it, and then clean up afterwards.

That's a lot of decisions and things that you're going to have to do in order to eat properly on this keto diet. That might not seem like a big deal as you're reading this. However, you can't think of things in the present moment when you're feeling good.

Imagine yourself after a long day at work. If you have children, you have to come home and take care of them. Are you going to feel like cooking and preparing a ketogenic meal 100% of the time in these situations?

For most people, the answer is probably no. And when you are on the ketogenic diet, all it takes is one mess up before you could potentially be on a slippery slope; it might take days or even weeks before you get back on track.

It's best to think of these things that might derail you from success in advance and plan for them ahead of time. That's essentially what the goal of meal prepping is, which is why it's so critical to your success on this diet plan in particular.

If you were following a different diet plan, maybe one that wasn't strict on how much protein, carbs, and fat you needed to eat, then meal prepping wouldn't matter as much. For example, let's say you're following a particular style of the 'if it fits your macros' diet that allows you to eat any foods you want as long as it fits within your macro percentages for the day.

And just so we're clear, I don't recommend following this style of the 'if it fits your macros' diet. However, for the sake of example, if you were following this diet plan, then meal prepping wouldn't be nearly as critical as it is on the ketogenic diet.

The reason for this is because you could easily eat fast food or processed foods quite often and still be on track with your diet plan. But in terms of the ketogenic diet, meal prepping will not only help to increase your chances of success on the diet, but it'll also help you save a lot of time.

By cooking in batches, you'll be saving time setting up to cook, and you'll also have fewer dishes to clean. Meal prepping can also save you money because you'll prepare the exact amount of food that you'll need to eat. you won't have to worry about wasting any of the excess.

Now that we've talked about some of the benefits to meal prepping, let's get into the actual process of how to go about doing it.

The Step-By-Step Process to Successfully Meal Prep on the Dirty Keto Diet

Here's the exact step-by-step process you need to follow in order to see success in regards to meal prepping on the ketogenic diet.

Step #1: Decide when it is that you want to meal prep

The first thing that you need to do is figure out when you want to meal prep. For most people, the best time to do this would be on a Sunday afternoon.

Usually, these days are going to be pretty relaxing and chill. You might not be doing anything on these days aside from watching sports, so you might as well prepare for the upcoming week while the games are on.

Of course, you're not limited to doing this on just Sundays. Depending on what your schedule is, a different day of the week might work better for you. The point is to try and meal prep on a day when you're off from work and you don't have much else going on.

If you don't want to meal prep on a single day, you can always split it up between two days. For example, on Sunday you could prep all of your meals for Monday, Tuesday, and Wednesday.

Then on Wednesday, you could prep your meals for the rest of the week. Be honest with yourself about how likely it is that you're going to stick to this regime.

If you're working a 9-to-5 job Monday through Friday, this would mean that you're going to have to plan and prepare for the rest of your meals on a day when you have to work.

If going to work gives you momentum to continue doing something productive for the rest of the day, then this could be a great option for you. However, if you know that you're likely not going to feel like doing much after work, then it's best to do all of your meal prepping on a single day when you're off from work.

I wouldn't recommend splitting up your meal prepping across more than two days. Anything more than that and it defeats the purpose of what we're trying to achieve in the first place.

Finally, you could meal prep during the mornings on the weekend if you're going to be waking up at the same time every day like I talked about in the chapter on sleep.

This would be a great way to maintain your new sleep schedule because you'd have something to do when you wake up. There's not a right or wrong time to choose when it comes to doing your meal prep. The main thing is that you're able to consistently do it, so pick a time when you're most likely to get the job done.

Step #2: Plan out all of your meals

This could be one of the more difficult steps in the process, however, it will get easier as time goes on. You'll be eating similar meals, and you'll know exactly what you need to buy and how to make it.

Initially, this can be a bit tedious. Remember though, this is something you would have to think about multiple times a day, and you'd have to make these decisions when you're mentally drained.

At least this way, you're fresh and you'll have an easier time making the correct decisions. The easiest way to go about doing this would be to use pen and paper or a spreadsheet.

You would write breakfast, lunch, and dinner going across the top row of the spreadsheet, and then you would write the days of the week going down the first column.

From here, you have a couple of different options as to what you can do. You can plan out all of your breakfasts for the week, then all of your lunches, followed by all of your dinners.

Or you can plan out all of your meals for Monday, then Tuesday, etc. Don't feel as if you need to eat 21 different meals over the course of the week. Keep things as simple as possible.

Initially, you might only want to try eating 2-3 different meals for breakfast as well as for lunch and dinner. For example, for breakfast, you might eat eggs and bacon on Monday. Then on Tuesday, you might make a cheddar cheese omelet.

And you'd simply rotate between eating these two breakfast meals throughout the week. This way you won't stress yourself out trying to think of different meals to eat.

And whether you are aware of this or not, people typically eat the same things more often than they realize. As time goes on, you can try out different meals; you're certainly not limited to the meals you can eat as long as they're keto approved.

Step #3: Work Out Your Macro Percentages

Steps 3 and 4 are interchangeable. You can do whichever one you prefer first. The benefit of calculating your macro percentages first is that you'll know exactly how much food you need to get at the grocery store.

On the other hand, if you go to the grocery store first, then you'll be estimating how much of certain foods you'll need. This, of course, isn't that big of a deal because if you're unsure, you can always buy more than you think you need. This would give you some leftovers for the following week.

Essentially though, what you need to do for this step is to figure out how much of each meal you're going to eat. Let's use the example of eating bacon and eggs for breakfast on Monday.

During this step, you need to figure out how many eggs it is that you're going to eat. Let's say you decide to eat 3 eggs. How are they going to be prepared? How much bacon are you going to eat?

These factors will affect the total caloric content and the macros. This is why it's a good idea to know ahead of time roughly how many calories it is that you want to consume per meal.

For example, if you're eating 2,000 calories a day, how do you want to break that up across your meals? You could do an even split between breakfast, lunch, and dinner, but you don't have to do that if you don't want to.

Some people (such as myself) prefer to eat smaller breakfasts and larger dinners. The reason why I personally like doing this is because breakfast isn't that social of a meal.

You're typically eating breakfast by yourself. With dinner though, you'll usually be eating that meal with friends or family, and it's more enjoyable if you can eat more calories.

If breakfast is an important meal in your household, you could always eat a large breakfast and a smaller dinner. It doesn't matter how you want to break up your calories across your meals. Simply do whatever will work best for you.

Once you've decided how many calories it is that you want to eat for each meal, you'll then have the framework you need to determine how much of certain foods you'll need to eat. Continuing on with our example of eating 2,000 calories per day, let's say the individual decides to split up his calories evenly across 3 meals.

This would mean that he's going to eat 667 calories per meal. In the case of eating bacon and eggs for breakfast, he could eat 4 fried eggs and 6 slices of bacon, assuming that each fried egg contains around 90 calories and each slice of bacon contains around 50 calories.

From here, all he would have to do is track how much fat and protein is contained in the eggs and bacon and he'd be good to go for this meal. Then on Tuesday, let's say he wants to eat the cheddar cheese omelet, and it's going to require 6 eggs to make.

If he's rotating between these two breakfast meals, then he knows that he'll need to get three dozen eggs to meal prep his breakfasts when he goes to the store to shop for his weekly groceries.

You would then repeat this process for lunch and dinner. After completing this process, you'd know exactly what it is that you need to get at the grocery store, which is why I recommend doing this step first before you buy your groceries.

Step #4: Buy your groceries

After you've determined what meals you're going to eat and how much of each food item you need, the next thing you need to do is go grocery shopping. If you're following things in the order I've outlined, all of the legwork has been done upfront.

Depending on what you're shopping for, you can buy in bulk or on a week to week basis. For example, different kinds of nuts you'll be eating on this dirty keto diet have long expiration dates.

You could buy these types of food items in bulk so that you always have some on hand, and you might be able to get a discount on them. However, most of the things you'll be buying will have short expiration dates.

This would include various things such as vegetables or dairy products. You're more than likely going to be better off buying these things on a week-to-week basis.

Buying in bulk when you can is great because it'll be that much less you have to shop for the following week. At the end of the day, shop in a manner that's easiest for you.

If grocery shopping once a week and getting the same things every time keeps things simple for you, then by all means do it. On the flip side, if you like buying in bulk, then do that whenever possible.

Step #5: Cook Your Meals

Now it's time for the fun part. You're going to cook and prepare your meals ahead of time. This will take a good chunk of your time, but there are some things you can do to save some time.

The first thing would be to start cooking the foods that will take the longest. For example, if there's some meat that needs to be slow-cooked, then go ahead and get that started first.

You can start preparing and cooking other things after you get that going. This'll help save you a lot of time because you don't want to wait until the end to start cooking something that's going to take 6 hours to finish.

The next tip is to cook in batches of individual ingredients when possible. For example, let's say one of your lunches is going to consist of a chicken salad with steamed broccoli, cheese, and olive oil for the dressing.

You don't have to prepare the broccoli and chicken in the same skillet. Instead, it's much easier to prepare all of the chicken that you're going to need for the week.

After you start preparing the chicken, you can separately prepare the other ingredients such as broccoli. Then once you're done, you'll be able to put the ingredients together for certain meals as needed.

Of course, this might not be possible for all of your meals. With certain meals on your calendar, you might not be able to add in ingredients later on. In these cases, go ahead and make everything together at once.

However, if you want to save some time, cook everything separately first and then combine ingredients later on whenever possible. The final tip is to be organized and have a plan ahead of time.

Know what it is that you need to get cooked and know the best order to cook it in. Whenever you have something baking in the oven, use that time to start cutting up vegetables or something else.

The better your plan of action, the smoother things will go. Know exactly what utensils, spices, oils, and other things you'll need and have them ready to go before you start. This can save you some time by preventing you from scrambling when you need something.

Step #6: Put Your Meals in Containers and Store Them

At this point, pat yourself on the back because most of the hard work has been done. Once everything has been cooked, you'll simply need to put all of your meals into meal prep containers and store them in a refrigerator.

As far as what kind of containers you should get, I recommend getting some nice glass meal prep containers. With glass containers, you don't have to worry about them containing any BPA's, and you won't have to worry about them not being microwave or dishwasher safe.

Of course, if you fear you might drop your containers, plastic isn't a bad option. Make sure you invest in some high-quality containers. You want these containers to last for a long time to come.

As long as the plastic containers are BPA free and microwave and dishwasher safe, then you'll be good to go. Some of the containers might even have separated compartments within them.

This is certainly handy depending on what meal you're eating, but it isn't necessary. Just go with whatever suits your particular needs best!

Finally, the last thing you'll want to make sure you do is label your containers. You don't want to have to look around and hunt down what you're going to eat for the day.

A simple label saying something like, "Monday's Breakfast", will easily suffice. This will help save you a lot of time.

The last thing you want is to be rushed in the morning and accidentally grab the wrong container before you head off to work. Labeling the containers will keep things clean and organized.

And as a side note, if you don't have enough room in your main refrigerator for all of these containers, then consider buying a mini fridge to store some or all of your prepped meals.

This is a great option if you have a family. You'll only have to worry about eating from your own fridge.

You won't be tempted by anything that's in the main fridge if your spouse isn't following a ketogenic diet. Hopefully you won't have to worry as much about your kids getting into your prepped meals either.

All in all though, make sure that you prepare in advance as much as you possibly can. Sticking to this diet plan isn't about having a lot of willpower, it's more about being prepared. If you can do that, then you'll be setting yourself up for a much greater chance of success.

Chapter 8: Building Muscle on a Dirty Ketogenic Diet

Throughout this book, I've talked about using the dirty ketogenic diet strictly for weight loss purposes. The majority of the people who are interested in the ketogenic diet want to follow it to lose weight.

However, your fitness goal may be different. You might be interested in building muscle, or maybe you want to lose some fat now and add some muscle down the line.

In this chapter, you're going to learn everything you need to know about building muscle on a ketogenic diet.

How Do Things Change When You Want to Build Muscle?

When you're trying to lose weight, the goal is to create a caloric deficit by burning off more calories than you consume. However, when you're trying to build muscle, you want to do the opposite.

You want to create a caloric surplus by eating more calories than you burn off. The reason for this is because you need to give your body enough of the raw materials it needs in order to pack on some new muscle.

Think of it like building a house. Let's say for the sake of example that you need 10,000 bricks to build a certain size house.

If your brick supplier is only able to supply you with 8,000 bricks, then the max-sized house you're going to be able to build is going to be smaller than you originally hoped for.

The same is true for your body. If your body needs 2,800 calories a day in order to maximize muscle gains, then if you don't eat that many calories you're going to be leaving muscle on the table.

Nutritionally, the amount of calories that you eat is the biggest difference between building muscle and burning fat. The other big difference between burning fat and building muscle is how you exercise.

If you're trying to burn fat, then you don't have to exercise at all if you don't want to. You can lose weight solely by following your diet plan.

Conversely, when it comes to building muscle you're going to need to do some form of resistance training. The reason for this is because you must provide your body with some sort of stimulus in order to build muscle.

If you're sedentary and eat more calories than you burn off, you'll just gain fat. Therefore, by working out, you'll be providing your body with a reason to grow back bigger and stronger.

Then once you combine working out with the right nutrition plan, you will start to build muscle. If you're interested in building muscle, the only thing that's going to change with the dirty keto diet is the total amount of calories that you're eating.

Everything else stays the same. Your macro percentages are the same, and the guidelines of what you can and can't eat stay the same, as well as everything else. The question now becomes how much you should eat in order to start building muscle.

How Many Calories Should You Eat to Build Muscle?

If you'll recall from an earlier chapter, we determined our resting metabolic rate which is the total number of calories someone burns per day by taking our current bodyweight and multiplying it by 13.

We're going to have the same starting point as if we're trying to burn fat. The difference is where we're going from that starting point.

Let's use an example of someone who currently weighs 200 pounds. He would take 200 and multiply that by 13 to get a total of 2,600.

This means that this individual burns off 2,600 calories in a given day. If he wanted to start losing weight he would need to eat less than this number.

However, if he wants to start building muscle, then he needs to eat more than this. The trick is to not eat way above this number.

The reason for this is because eating too many calories can lead to excess fat gain. We essentially want to eat enough to build muscle, but not too much to the point where we gain fat.

The best way to strike this balance is to aim to gain half a pound a week. This means that you'll need to add 250 calories to your resting metabolic rate because it takes a surplus of roughly 3,500 calories to gain one pound.

Continuing on with our example, this person would take his resting metabolic rate of 2,600 and add 250 to it to get a total of 2,850.

Therefore, this person would need to eat 2,850 calories per day in order to gain half a pound of muscle per week. Once this step is done, the next thing you need to do is calculate your macro percentages.

As I mentioned earlier, the percentages of fat, protein, and carbs that you're going to eat stay the same, regardless of whether the goal is to build muscle or to burn fat.

This means we're still going to eat 75% of our total calories from fat, 20% from protein, and the remaining 5% from carbs. Here's a breakdown of what that looks like:

2,850 x 0.75= 2,137.5 calories per day from fat
2,850 x 0.2= 570 calories per day from protein
2,850 x 0.05= 142.5 calories per day from carbs

We can then determine the gram equivalent by doing the following:

2,137.5/9 = 237.5 grams of fat per day
570/4 = 142.5 grams of protein per day
142.5/4 = 35.6 grams of carbs per day

From here all you have to do is stay on track with your calories and macros, and you'll be good to go. You don't have to worry about changing any of the fundamentals of the dirty keto diet when your primary goal is to build muscle.

Workout You Can Use to Build Muscle

The last thing I want to leave you with before I wrap up this chapter is a muscle-building workout that you can do at the gym. It's a very simple routine, but that doesn't mean it's ineffective.

As long as you focus on increasing the amount of weight you lift over time, then you'll be good to go. Here's the workout:

Monday: Push Workout

- Incline Dumbbell Bench Press—3 sets of 6 reps, 2 minutes rest between sets
- Standing Dumbbell Military Press—3 sets of 8 reps, 90 seconds rest between sets
- Standing Dumbbell Lateral Raises—3 sets of 10 reps, 60 seconds rest between sets
- Tricep Rope Pushdowns—3 sets of 12 reps, 60 seconds rest between sets
- Tricep Dumbbell Kickbacks—3 sets of 12 reps, 60 seconds rest between sets

Wednesday: Pull Workout

- Lat Pulldowns—3 sets of 8 reps, 90 seconds rest between sets
- Chest Supported Dumbbell Row—3 sets of 8 reps, 90 seconds rest between sets
- Bent Over Flys with Dumbbells—3 sets of 12 reps, 60 seconds rest between sets
- Standing Barbell Curls—3 sets of 8 reps, 90 seconds rest between sets
- Incline Dumbbell Curls—3 sets of 10 reps, 60 seconds rest between sets

Friday: Leg Workout

- Goblet Squats—3 sets of 8 reps, 90 seconds rest between sets

- Leg Press—3 sets of 8 reps, 90 seconds rest between sets
- Leg Extensions—3 sets of 10 reps, 60 seconds rest between sets
- Hamstring Curls—3 sets of 10 reps, 60 seconds rest between sets
- Standing Calf Raises—3 sets of 15 reps, 45 seconds rest between sets

Note: A rep is one complete motion of an exercise and a set is a series of repetitions. For example, on the standing barbell curl exercise, you're doing the movement for 3 sets of 8 reps per set.

One single rep of the exercise would be you curling the bar upwards from resting on your thighs towards your shoulders. Then you would control the bar on the way back down to the starting position.

Once the barbell returns to the starting position, that completes one rep. You'd complete that movement 7 more times for a total of 8 reps.

Once you reach 8 reps, you would then take the prescribed amount of rest time, which in this case is 90 seconds. After the rest period is up, you would then perform another 8 reps, which would complete set number 2.

You would rest another 90 seconds before completing your final set consisting of 8 repetitions. After the third set, you would then move on and start the next exercise.

Chapter 9: Frequently Asked Questions

What Kinds of Foods Should I Eat on a Dirty Ketogenic Diet?

You might be wondering what some good food choices are for this diet plan. Here are some good ideas for fat, protein, and carb sources:

Protein:

- Lean meats such as chicken, beef, venison, turkey, etc.
- Fish
- Eggs
- Cottage cheese

Fat:

- Eggs
- Avocados
- Olive and coconut oil
- Flax and chia seeds
- Various nuts such as pecans and macadamia nuts
- Cheese

Carbs:

- Kale
- Spinach
- Broccoli
- Cauliflower

- Berries such as raspberries and blackberries due to their low net carbs. (Always be sure to check that they fit within your macros.)

Spices:

- Rosemary
- Pink Himalayan salt
- Black pepper
- Oregano
- Basil

This isn't a comprehensive list by any means. These are just some ideas to get you started. As long as you're eating a high amount of fat, a moderate amount of protein, and a low amount of carbs, then you'll be good to go.

What Are Some Popular Foods People Think Are Keto Approved But Aren't?

This is definitely something you want to think about before you start the dirty keto plan. You don't want to regularly eat something you think is keto approved when in reality, it isn't. Here are some popular foods people think are okay to eat on a keto diet, but aren't in reality:

Carrots: you might think that carrots are okay to eat on a ketogenic diet because they're a vegetable, and vegetables are good for you. While that certainly is the case, that doesn't mean that all vegetables are acceptable on certain diet plans.

The reality is that carrots contain too much sugar and have too many net carbs for them to be acceptable on this diet plan. Most leafy green vegetables contain a lot of fiber, making their net carbs zero or very close to it.

This allows you to eat as many of these kinds of vegetables as you please and not have the worry about getting kicked out of ketosis. The same can't be said for carrots, so it's best to avoid them altogether.

Fruit: this can be another tricky food item for some people to wrap their mind around as to why it's not okay to eat. Our whole lives, we've been told that fruit is good for us due to the rich amount of vitamins and nutrients that they contain.

While this may be true, that doesn't mean that fruit is good for you on certain diet plans. On the dirty ketogenic diet plan, fruit isn't going to do you any favors.

It contains a high amount of fructose, which will kick you out of ketosis. The only real exception to this are raspberries and blackberries.

These berries specifically contain a low enough amount of net carbs that you can enjoy some from time to time and not have to worry about getting kicked out of ketosis.

Certain Nuts Such as Cashews and Walnuts: Not all nuts are keto approved, and the main reason for this is because some nuts contain a high amount of net carbs. Cashews are the worst nut that you can eat on a ketogenic diet because they contain the highest amount of net carbs.

Walnuts also contain a good amount of net carbs, although it's not quite as high as cashews. Almonds could also be included on this list, even though they are low enough in net carbs for you to be able to enjoy some from time to time.

Almonds are probably one of the most popular nuts that exist, but they're overrated, especially on a ketogenic diet. They contain a higher amount of net carbs than other nuts, and they contain a high amount of Omega 6 fatty acids.

This type of fat acts as in inflammatory in the body, and most people need to improve the ratio of Omega 3's (which acts as an anti-inflammatory) to Omega 6's in their diet.

Almonds simply won't help you out in that regard. However, the overall amount of net carbs is low enough to where you could have some here and there if you really wanted to. At the end of the day though, there are simply some better choices out there when it comes to nuts.

Am I Allowed to Drink Alcohol on the Dirty Ketogenic Diet?

For the most part, you're going to be very limited on what you can have as far as alcohol is concerned on the ketogenic diet. Most beers are going to contain too many carbs, which will kick you out of ketosis.

However, there are some light beers that you could have. You'll definitely want to check and see what the carb content is before you start to drink though.

Depending on what your overall calories are, you most likely would be able to have 1-2 light beers and be fine. Wine is similar to beer in this regard.

Most wines are going to contain too much sugar for it to be okay on a ketogenic diet. Even with this being the case though, you can have dry wine and be fine. Other alcoholic beverages that are acceptable on a ketogenic diet are whiskey, dry martinis, and plain vodka.

Again though, the main thing you want to be sure you do is to check and see how much sugar these beverages contain before you drink them. In the case of vodka for example, most of the time it's flavored, and the flavoring will add a bunch of sugar, which makes it bad for a ketogenic diet.

And even if you're consuming something such as a light beer, this doesn't mean that you have permission to go crazy.

Remember that you're still only allowed to eat 5% of your total calories from carbs.

Any alcohol you consume still has to fit within that. As long as you follow that rule and stick within the parameters of your macros, then you'll be good to go.

Can I Build Muscle and Burn Fat at the Same Time?

You might be interested in burning fat and building muscle. So is it possible to do both at the same time?

My answer to that would be that it depends. If someone already has a lot of muscle to begin with and is pretty lean, then it would be extremely hard for that individual to do both at the same time.

He would be much better off focusing on one goal at a time. On the other hand, if there's someone who's completely new to weightlifting and he has quite a bit of body fat to lose, then yes, it's certainly possible to burn fat and build muscle at the same time.

The thing is that you don't want to get caught up trying to chase two rabbit holes. It's better to focus on one goal at a time.

For example, if you have some extra fat to lose, but you also want to build some muscle, then focus solely on burning fat. The reality is that as a beginner, you can focus on burning fat and still build some muscle if you're lifting weights.

While it's technically possible to build muscle while you're in a caloric deficit, it's not optimal, which is why the advanced trainee would need to be in a caloric surplus in order to pack on some new size.

That's why it's best to focus on one goal at a time, and after achieving that goal, move onto the next goal and focus solely on that. For example, if someone currently weighs 200 pounds, he could lose the excess weight and get down to 170 pounds.

Then once he reaches that number, he could focus purely on building muscle. He could build 10 pounds of muscle to reach a bodyweight of 180. Think of any muscle you gain while you're trying to burn fat as a cool bonus and nothing more.

Don't go out of your way to try and make both happen at the same time because that could cause you to not achieve either goal.

How Can I Tell if I'm in the State of Ketosis?

The best way to know if you're in a state of ketosis or not is to test, test, test. There are a couple of different ways you can go about doing this.

The first method is to use urine test strips. Essentially you'll dip the test strip in a sample of your urine. Then after waiting roughly 15 seconds, a purplish color should start to appear on the strip.

A darker color of purple indicates a higher level of ketosis. A lighter shade of purple indicates lower levels of ketosis.

The key with the urine strips is to make sure that you have a consistent level of hydration when you take the test. You don't want to be dehydrated or super hydrated when you take the test.

Either of these two things can result in a false reading on the test. Instead, aim for your urine to have a slight yellow color to it and you should be good to go.

The other way you can test to see if you're in ketosis or not is to use a blood test. This is going to be a bit more expensive than the urine test strips, however, it's easier to get a more accurate and consistent reading.

You'll simply prick your finger and get an instant reading on the amount of ketones in your blood. Most of these test kits will come with a chart that'll show you if you currently have high or low levels of ketosis.

Finally, if you don't want to spend money on test kits, then there are some signs you can look out for to see if you're entering into a state of ketosis. These signs and symptoms are the same ones you'll experience if you get the keto flu.

These are things such as weakness, fatigue, headaches, nausea, and brain fog, among other things. However, if you're following the recommendations I outlined in the chapter on the keto flu, then it's possible that you might greatly lessen or even prevent the onset of the symptoms to begin with.

That's why using these symptoms to gauge if you're entering into a state of ketosis or not can be tricky. Not only that, but let's say you get into ketosis and then later on down the line you eat more carbs than you should have.

You're not sure if you ate too many carbs to kick you out of ketosis. The only way you'd be able to tell if you did get kicked out of ketosis is if you test for it.

Once you test for it, you can confirm whether or not you did indeed get kicked out of ketosis. After this, you can test along the way to know when you get back into ketosis.

What Are Some Examples of Things I Can Have on a Dirty Keto Diet that Aren't Allowed on a Standard Keto Diet?

On a normal ketogenic diet, everything you eat needs to be wholesome (i.e. natural) and organic when possible. On a dirty ketogenic diet, you don't have to follow that. You can essentially eat what you want as long as it contains a low amount of carbs, and you're still on track to hit your daily protein and fat macros.

This means that you can eat certain things such as processed foods, fast food, and drinks that contain artificial sweeteners. An example of this might be getting a bacon, egg, and cheese breakfast sandwich from a fast food restaurant.

You obviously wouldn't be able to eat the English muffin part of it, but everything else would be approved on a dirty ketogenic diet. However, on a strict or standard ketogenic diet, this breakfast item wouldn't be approved because of how it's been processed and prepared.

Another example would be something such as pork rinds. It's fine on a dirty keto diet, but because it's a processed food, it isn't approved on the standard keto diet.

So since this is a dirty keto diet, does that mean you can go crazy and eat whatever processed foods you want, whenever you want? Well, look at the next question for the answer to that...

How Should I Balance Eating Processed Foods with Clean Wholesome Foods?

Even though you technically could eat nothing but processed foods, that doesn't mean that you should. The reason for this is because you won't feel as good energy-wise if you eat nothing but junk food.

These foods items also contain a higher amount of calories in general than wholesome foods do. This is definitely something you'll want to think about because you're overall calories are going to be restricted since you're trying to lose weight.

Finally, wholesome foods such as vegetables are high in fiber, which is something that'll help you stay fuller for a longer period of time. You'll definitely want to take advantage of that when you're on a weight loss diet.

On the flip side, you don't want to eat clean foods all of the time either. This can make the diet plan hard to keep up with for the long haul. It could also make it more likely that you'll cheat on the diet, feel guilty, and then binge eat.

So there does need to be a proper balance between the two. The best way I've found to hit that balance is to eat clean wholesome foods 85% of the time. For the remaining 15% of the time, eat the processed foods that are allowed on the dirty ketogenic diet.

This allows you to enjoy certain food items you like from time to time, but it's not enough to make you feel sick from all of the junk food and potentially ruin the diet plan.

Remember that it's not what you eat 15% of the time that causes health problems—it's what you eat the majority of the time that can ruin your health. If you like eating pork rinds for example, and that helps to keep you moving forward, then by all means do it.

You just have to do so in the right amount. Eating an entire bag of pork rinds every single day would be too extreme, even for a dirty keto diet.

Having some from time to time is perfectly fine. As long as you strike a balance, you'll be good to go. And the best way to go about doing that is to eat natural foods 85% of the time and non-wholesome keto-approved foods the remaining 15% of the time.

Conclusion

You now have everything you need in order to be successful with this dirty keto diet plan. All that's left for you to do is execute on the plan.

There will certainly be some bumps in the road, but as long as you stay strong and persistent, you'll make it to your end destination. This diet plan will work as long as you stick to it.

If you give up and quit, then you won't be able to achieve your goal. Therefore, stick with it during good times and bad times. It'll be well worth it, so don't give up!

Did you enjoy reading this book? If so, please consider leaving a review. Even just a few words would help others decide if the book is right for them.

Best regards and thanks in advance—Thomas

Sources

(1) https://www.ncbi.nlm.nih.gov/pubmed/22825659

(2) https://www.ncbi.nlm.nih.gov/pubmed/14596707

(3) https://www.ncbi.nlm.nih.gov/pmc/articles/PMC4434546/

Endomorph Diet

Strategically Use Intermittent Fasting and Flexible Dieting to Work with Your Body Type

Thomas Rohmer

Copyright © 2018

Rohmerfitness All rights reserved.

No part of this publication may be reproduced, distributed, or
transmitted in any form or by any means, including photocopying, recording, or other electronic or mechanical methods, without the prior written permission and consent of the publisher, except in the in the case of brief quotations embodied in product reviews and certain other noncommercial uses permitted by copyright law.

Disclaimer:

This guide has been created for informational and reference purposes only. The author, publisher, and any other affiliated parties cannot be held in any way accountable for any personal injuries or damage allegedly resulting from the information contained herein, or from any misuse of such guidance. Although strict measures have been taken to provide accurate information, the parties involved with the creation and publication of this guide take no responsibility for any issues that may arise from alleged discrepancies contained herein. It is strongly recommended that you consult a physician, personal trainer, and nutritionist prior to commencing this or any other workout or diet plan. This guide is not a substitute for professional personal guidance from a qualified medical professional. If you feel pain or discomfort at any point during exercises contained herein, cease the activity immediately and seek medical guidance.

Before You Begin:

Get the Latest Scoop on the Most Cutting Edge Info on Health & Fitness!

As thanks for picking up this book, I'd love to offer you the chance to maximize your results by getting exclusive info on health and fitness.

You'll be the first to know when I publish new books, and you'll receive exclusive content on health and fitness that I only share with people on my list.

Simply visit the link directly below and get started on the path to the healthiest version of yourself today!

https://rohmerfitness.lpages.co/kindle-sign-up/

Table Of Contents

Chapter 1: Why the Struggle is Real as an Endomorph..120
Chapter 2: Why the Game Plan Needs to Change if You Want to See Success...123
Chapter 3: The Endomorph Diet Plan..................132
Chapter 4: Why Me? The Correct Endomorph Mindset You Need to Have.....................................149
Chapter 5: Endomorph Exercise—How to Workout in a Way That's Optimal for Your Body Type........165
Chapter 6: What You Need to Do to Ensure the Weight Stays Off...181
Chapter 7: Endomorph Supplement Guide..........186
Chapter 8: Frequently Asked Questions...............210

Introduction

Life gives us challenges, that's for sure. Everyone has his or her ups and downs in life.

Your current struggles might be in regards to your body type. If you're an endomorph, it can almost seem unfair that you were born with such a body type.

It can especially seem this way when you look at other people like ectomorphs, people who can seemingly eat whatever they want and not gain a pound. Sure, you may not have been born with a lightning-fast metabolism like they were, but that doesn't mean all hope is lost.

In fact, being an endomorph isn't all bad; there are actually some advantages to it, contrary to what you might believe. Still, this doesn't take away from the fact that losing weight and keeping it off can be a big-time struggle for endomorphs.

Therefore, specific strategies must be taken in order to achieve lasting results. Regular diet and exercise advice simply won't cut it.

And in this book, I'm going to share with you what you need to be doing differently as an endomorph in order to help you achieve your health and fitness goals.

Also before we get into the nitty gritty of the book please consider leaving a review if you enjoy it. Even just a few words will help other people know if the book is right for them. Many thanks in advance! Now let's dive in!

Chapter 1: Why the Struggle is Real as an Endomorph

Do you feel like you gain weight just by looking at food sometimes? Almost as if it doesn't matter how little you eat because that food still seems to get stored as body fat?

This is why being an endomorph is a real struggle. Endomorphs have slower metabolisms, which can make it harder for their bodies to burn off the calories from the foods that they eat.

Don't worry though, this book will help you to implement strategies that will help you increase your metabolism over time, and teach you to eat in a way that won't allow your metabolism to destroy any hope you have for success. I'm not saying you'll develop the metabolism of an ectomorph, but improvement is what we're looking to achieve.

There are three main body types—ectomorph, mesomorph, and endomorph. Here's a breakdown of the differences between the three:

Ectomorph: characterized by a smaller bone structure with smaller ankles and wrists. Taller individuals tend to be ectomorphs. They usually have really fast metabolisms and struggle to put on muscle more so than the other two body types.

Mesomorph: a mesomorph is someone in the middle of an ectomorph and endomorph. Most people consider this to be the ideal body type to have because mesomorphs put on muscle easier than ectomorphs, and they don't gain fat as easily as an endomorph does. Metabolism wise, they're right in the middle. Their metabolism isn't nearly as fast as a typical ectomorph, but it's not as slow as an endomorph.

Endomorph: characterized as someone who is stockier and has a larger bone structure—meaning larger ankles and wrists. Endomorphs tend to store fat easily and have lower muscle definition due to the extra adipose tissue. Endomorphic bodies typically use sugar for fuel more so than fat, hence why it can be harder to burn fat. Finally, endomorphs tend to have the slowest metabolism of any of the body types, but building muscle tends to come easier than it does for ectomorphs.

How can I tell if I'm Truly an Endomorph?

Right now you may not totally be sure if you're an endomorph or not. Just because someone is overweight doesn't automatically mean that they're an endomorph.

For example, an ectomorph might suffer from what is commonly referred to as skinny fat syndrome. This is when a person has a low level of muscle mass and also has a higher level of body fat, which makes the stomach stick out.

A person like this would still be classified as an ectomorph who needs to drop the body fat and add some muscle mass in order to solve the problem. With that being said, the easiest way to tell what body type you are is to do the following test—take your thumb and middle finger and wrap them around your opposing wrist.

If your middle finger and thumb don't wrap around fully to touch each other, then you're an endomorph. If you're thumb and middle finger wrap around perfectly to just be touching each other, then you're a mesomorph.

And finally, if your thumb and index finger overlap each other, then you're an ectomorph.

Hopefully, you know now if you're an endomorph or not. And if you are, don't worry.

This book will help give you the strategies that you need in order to succeed. It can be easy to play the blame-game or wonder why you were born a certain way.

However, as you'll see in the coming chapters, wishing to be born with better genetics ultimately won't change anything. Having the right attitude is critical in being able to overcome your weight loss struggles.

Yes, you have more difficult challenges ahead then other people might due to your body type. However, looking at others and comparing yourself to them won't do you the least bit of good.

You have no idea where they're starting from, what they've been through, or what they've done in order for them to get to where they are today. The key here is to focus on yourself and not compare.

I'm going to give you all of the tools you need in order to succeed (not just with diet and exercise but mindset as well), but ultimately, it's still up to you to put these plans into action to get results.

Chapter 2: Why the Game Plan Needs to Change if You Want to See Success

For some people, losing weight comes quite easily. For you though, you might have to work a bit harder at it in order to see success.

What works for one person may not work for you as an endomorph. That's why you're going to need a different game plan from someone else whose body type makes it easier for him or her to get in better shape.

Before we get into the specifics of how things need to change, let's first cover the basic principles of fat loss...

How Does Your Body Burn Fat?

In order to understand the best game plan, it's first important for you to understand how your body actually burns fat. Most people don't know this, but it really isn't that complicated.

Everyday your body has functions that it must maintain, such as breathing and digesting food. These processes require energy in order to continue functioning.

So where do our bodies get the energy it needs in order to continue functioning? It comes from the foods that we eat.

The foods we eat contain energy (i.e. calories), and that energy is then used to help fuel our bodies to move, breathe, and digest food, among many other things. Our bodies only need a certain amount of energy in order to maintain all of these processes.

If you consume more energy than your body needs, the rest will get stored as fat. This is known as a caloric surplus.

On the other hand, if you consume fewer calories than your body needs, it'll tap into your fat stores to get the remaining energy it needs to continuing functioning. This is known as the caloric deficit.

The total amount of energy your body needs in a given day is known as your resting metabolic rate (RMR for short). In other words, your resting metabolic rate is the total amount of calories your body burns off in a given day.

Here's a breakdown of everything I just described:

Mike's resting metabolic rate is 2,300 calories. This means that he burns off 2,300 calories each and every day. Therefore:

- If Mike eats more than 2,300 calories per day, he'll be in a caloric surplus and start to gain weight.
- If Mike eats less than 2,300 calories per day, he'll be in a caloric deficit and start to lose weight.
- If Mike eats right at 2,300 calories per day, he'll be at his maintenance calories and he'll maintain his current bodyweight.

Therefore, if you want to start losing weight you must burn off more calories than you consume. Always remember this!

Every diet that's ever been created has always had the goal of getting you to consume fewer calories in one way or another in order to put you into a caloric deficit. Now some ways are better than others of course.

Most mainstream diets today are set up to make you fail before you even start. And as an endomorph, we need to be strategic with our approach in how we're going to go about creating a caloric deficit.

How Do You Calculate Your Resting Metabolic Rate?

The first step that we need to take is to figure out how many calories it is that you burn off in a given day. The calculation for this is quite simple.

All you need to do is take your current bodyweight and multiply it by 13—that's your RMR. Let's use me as an example:

Current bodyweight=210

210x13=2,730

This means that I burn off 2,730 calories per day. I'll need to start eating less than that if I want to start losing weight.

The question then becomes, how large of a caloric deficit should you create in order to start losing weight? If you create too large of a deficit, you'll be hungry all of the time and eventually crash and burn.

On the flip side, if you create too small of a deficit, then it'll take way too long for you to reach your goal. You want to land somewhere in the middle of these two extremes.

The best way to do that is to aim to lose around one pound of fat per week. At first glance, that might not seem like a lot, however keep in mind that I'm talking about pure fat loss here.

I'm not talking about losing water weight or anything like that. Losing even 5 pounds of pure fat can make a big difference in how you look.

Imagine one year from now being 52 pounds lighter. It's very possible to do if you go about doing things in the right manner and focus on long-term results rather than quick fixes.

Quick fixes are what most people do when they go on a crash diet to lose 20 pounds in a month. The problem is that these diets are too extreme and people end up going back to their old eating patterns.

And when that happens, so does rebound weight gain. So how much should you eat in order to burn one pound of fat per week?

There are approximately 3,500 calories in one pound of fat (1). This means that you need to create an average weekly caloric deficit of 3,500 calories in order to burn one pound of fat.

Take 3,500 and divide it by 7 days in the week and that comes out to an average daily deficit of 500 calories per day. Let's continue using myself as an example:

Resting metabolic rate: 2,730

2,730-500=2,230

This means that I need to consume 2,230 calories per day in order to start burning off one pound of fat per week.

Remember though, the goal is to create a weekly caloric deficit of 3,500 calories. That means that you could create a larger caloric deficit on some days and a smaller caloric deficit on other days.

For example, if it's a Saturday and you know that you might go out for dinner with your family, you could create a deficit that's smaller than 500 calories. Let's say you create a deficit of 250 calories; this will allow you to enjoy a meal at a restaurant with your family.

Then on a different day, maybe a Tuesday when you don't have much going on, you could create a larger deficit of 750 calories to make up for the smaller deficit. The point is that you can break up things however you please as long as you create an average deficit of 3,500 calories over the course of the week.

If it makes things easier for you to do a 500-calorie deficit every day, then stick with that. However, don't think that you have to create the same sized deficit every day because you certainly don't.

Now that you know how your body burns fat, and you know how many calories you need to eat to start losing weight, let's get into more specifics about what to do diet-wise in order to start burning fat.

Diet Game Plan to Lose Weight as an Endomorph

The body's first source of energy is carbs. Our bodies use carbs for fuel before it taps into our fat stores.

That's true regardless of what body type you are. However, you may have noticed that, as an endomorph, your body may struggle more to burn off carbs, and thus your body is never given the chance to use fat for fuel.

You might have eaten carbs late at night right before bed and then felt like you gained a couple of pounds the next morning. The reason for this is because when we eat food, our insulin levels increase.

Insulin is a hormone that allows glucose from the carbohydrates you eat to enter into cells so that they can be used for energy. The kicker is that the extra glucose will then get converted into lipids and stored as fat for later use.

Not only does insulin signal the body to store fat, but insulin also inhibits the breakdown of fat. This means that your body doesn't burn fat when insulin levels are high.

Essentially, if you're eating a heavy carbohydrate meal right before bed, your body is busy breaking those carbs you just ate down into glucose. Then your body is taking that glucose and putting it into cells and storing the excess as fat instead of burning fat.

This is why one of the strategies we're going to implement is to limit our carbohydrate intake. Notice I said limit, not eliminate.

I want this diet plan to be something that you can do for the rest of your life. If we completely got rid of carbs, then you wouldn't ever be able to enjoy your favorite salty or sugary treats.

Yes, you can still eat foods like chocolate chip cookies and potato chips, and still lose weight if you go about doing it in the right manner, which I'll show you how to do in a later chapter. Carbohydrates aren't the problem in and of itself.

The problem is eating an excessive amount of carbs. Many people act as if carbs are the root of the obesity epidemic, but they're not.

Overeating in general and a lack of exercise is a far more likely cause. Right now though, I want you to understand that if around 50% of your total caloric intake is coming from carbs, than that's too high.

We're going to need to scale that back some so that you can give your body a chance to use fat for fuel instead of carbs. We're going to replace the excess carbs with more protein and fat, which are more satiating than carbs.

This will allow you to stay fuller for a longer period of time while consuming fewer calories overall. This is very important since you're calories are going to be restricted in order to start losing weight.

The next thing we're going to implement is an intermittent fasting protocol. Fasting is essentially where you take a break from eating for a certain period of time.

For example, you might fast for 16 hours of the day and then eat during the remaining 8 hours of the day. I'll explain the exact plan in more detail in the following chapter, but for now, know that the lower carb intake combined with fasting is going to create a powerful fat-burning effect.

I already mentioned why decreasing carb intake is going to be important, but how will fasting help you out? Fasting will define when you can and can't eat.

So for example, if you're fasting for 16 hours a day, you might consume your first meal at noon and your last meal at 8:00 p.m. Then after 8:00 p.m. you'll be fasting for 16 hours until noon again the next day.

This is much better than consuming breakfast soon after you wake up. Breakfast is a lie that we've all been fed from a young age.

We've all been told things such as "breakfast is the most important meal of the day," or "make sure that you eat a big healthy breakfast so you can do well on your test at school today."

Wrong! Wrong! Wrong! Breakfast isn't the most important meal of the day, it's simply a meal, just like any other.

The point of eating is to give our bodies fuel to continue functioning. Therefore, we need to eat when our bodies need fuel.

We don't need to eat because it's a certain time of the day. You're also dehydrated when you first wake up.

Have you ever heard someone tell you that the water you drink at the start of the day is the most important water you'll drink all day? Of course not, that's ridiculous!

You drink water to hydrate your body. It doesn't matter *when* you drink water, what matters is that you hydrate your body when your body is in need of water.

This lie of breakfast has been perpetuated by cereal companies. They needed some way to promote their new breakfast cereals.

And by saying breakfast was the most important meal of the day, they were able to get everyone to buy into this idea that breakfast really was a meal more important than others. On top of that, they would coat their cereals with sugar, preservatives, and other additives to make us hooked on it.

Then we would have to keep coming back for more. Our ancestors didn't eat breakfast.

In fact, they ate more intermittently, similar to what you'll be doing with the fasting plan. They didn't have the luxury of waking up, walking to their fridge, taking out some milk, and then eating a bowl of cereal.

Instead, they had to hunt for their food. Sometimes it would be a while before they found a herd of animals to hunt and feast on.

And if they didn't find any food, they'd of course be fasting in the meantime. So rather than starting your day off with some sugary cereal that's going to spike your insulin and make it harder for you to burn fat, you're instead going to be skipping breakfast.

This will give your body more time to be in a fasted state because you won't be consuming any calories until later on in the day. This'll allow your insulin levels to stay at a low baseline level, giving your body more time to burn fat.

For some people who are looking to lose weight, these strategies may not be necessary. There are plenty of ways to lose weight.

However, as an endomorph, this lower carb and intermittent fasting strategy will help to give you the best chance of success because it works with your body type and not against it.

Chapter 3: The Endomorph Diet Plan

Now it's time for the fun part. We're going to get into the specifics of the diet plan that you need to do in order to start losing weight. I made this into a step-by-step format to make it easy to follow along with:

Step 1: Know How Many Calories It Is That You Need to Eat

We determined this in the previous chapter, but as a quick reminder, take your current bodyweight and multiply it by 13. Then take that number and subtract 500 from it.

For example, if you currently weigh 250 pounds, you would multiply that by 13 and get 3,250. You would then subtract 500 from 3,250 for a total of 2,750.

This is how many calories you need to eat on a daily basis in order to start losing one pound of fat per week.

Step 2: Determine Your Macros

A macronutrient is something your body needs in large quantities in order to sustain life. The three macronutrients are protein, carbs, and fat.

The next step we need to take in our diet plan is to figure out what percentage of our diet protein, carbs, and fat will each consist of. Here's a breakdown of the macro percentages you need to eat:

- Protein - 40%
- Fat - 35%
- Carbs - 25%

You'll notice that's still a fair amount of carbs. It's not a crazy low amount such as 5%, but it's also not high enough to ruin the diet.

This way, you'll still get to enjoy your favorite foods that are carbs. This will help set you up for long-term success instead of quitting and binge eating when the diet gets too hard.

Now we must convert these macro percentages into calories as part of our overall plan. Let's continue using myself as an example.

Recall from earlier that we figured out that I need to consume 2,730 calories per day in order to start losing one pound of fat per week.

Here's how to calculate how much protein, carbs, and fat I need to be consuming based on the percentages from above:

- 2,730x.4=1,092 calories from protein each day
- 2,730x.35=955.5 calories from fat each day
- 2,730x.25=682.5 calories from carbs each day

I can then determine how many grams this equates to by doing the following:

- 1,092/4= 273 grams of protein per day
- 955.5/9= 106.2 grams of fat per day
- 682.5/4= 170.63 grams of carbs per day

Once you've calculated these numbers, it's time to move onto the next step...

Step 3: Track All of the Calories and Macros that You Consume

I'll discuss what to eat in more depth later on, but one of the first things you want to make sure that you're doing is tracking the calories and macros that you eat. You may be surprised to realize just how many calories are in the common foods that we eat.

Most people underestimate how many calories they eat. This causes a big problem—you won't be losing any weight because you're eating more than you think you are!

That's why you must track how many calories it is that you're eating to ensure you're heading in the right direction. Yes, this can be tedious at times, but remember, if you want results that others don't have, you have to be willing to do what others won't do.

And thanks to modern technology, it's not that bad. Simply use your smartphone and download a macro tracking app.

Most of them have similar features and will easily be able to do what you need it for. Once you've downloaded the app, you're simply going to log anything that you eat into the app.

Yes, this also means that you're going to need to log any drinks you consume that contain calories as well. You can type in the foods that you eat into the app, and it'll be able to track how many calories it contains as well as the protein, carb, and fat content.

Most of the apps even have a barcode scanner, which allows you to easily be able to scan the foods you're eating and automatically log the information. One important thing that you'll want to make sure you get right is the portion sizes.

For example, the app obviously won't know how much steak you're eating. That's why it's important to carefully check food labels and measure out your food portions, even using a food scale if necessary.

Sometimes you'll find yourself in a tricky situation. For example, you might be at a restaurant and notice that the nutritional information isn't listed online or on the menu.

If that's the case, you'll want to use the eyeball test in situations such as these. Essentially, you're going to take your best guess as to how many calories are contained within the meal that you're eating.

You'll get better with this as time goes on, so don't sweat too much if you're not sure how many calories something contains. The best rule of thumb to go by when you're guesstimating is to always err on the side of more calories, not less.

This way you won't accidentally overeat and stall your progress. And finally, don't worry about hitting your numbers spot on each and every day.

I'd go nuts if I had to measure and eat exactly 170.63 grams of carbs per day. Get within 5% of the numbers I recommend and you'll be good to go.

Some days, things might work out to where you ate 30% of your total calories from carbs. Other days it might turn out to be 20%. Overall as long as your carbohydrate intake averages out to around 25% or so, you'll be good to go.

Step 4: Implement the Fasting Protocol

Now that you know how many calories, protein, carbs, and fat you need to eat, the next thing you need to do is add in the intermittent fasting protocol. Fasting is going to provide the framework for when to eat.

There are many different styles of intermittent fasting that exist today. Different ones work great for different people.

For example, some people really like to do longer fasts where they might fast for 24-36 hours straight 1-2 times per week. I'm not the biggest fan of these fasting methods for one simple reason—lack of consistency.

Since you're only doing these fasts 1-2 times per week, this can make it harder for your body to get used to fasting. Not only that, but depending on the situation you find yourself in on that day, you might skip the fast all together!

Let's say you do a 36-hour fast starting on Wednesday leading into Thursday. Your friend invites you to dinner to celebrate his birthday that night.

You don't want to turn him down, so you say yes with the caveat that you'll start the fast on Thursday instead. Now you're out of your normal routine and chances are good that you might not even get around to doing that fast.

Imagine if you wanted to try a new sleep schedule where you slept for 11 hours a day 5 days of the week and 30 minutes the other two days of the week. How hard do you think it would be for your body to adapt to that sleeping schedule?

It would be extremely difficult! You could make things much easier on yourself by sleeping a consistent 8 hours each and every night.

That's why I like fasting routines that are more consistent on a day-to-day basis. For example, some fasting protocols have you fasting every day.

This might sound extreme at first, but it's actually way easier to do because you're giving your body a consistent pattern of eating that it can adapt to. And since you're fasting every day, you won't have to fast as long.

Ideally, you'd fast for 16 hours every day; however depending on what your schedule is, fasting for only 14 hours is acceptable as well. Here's a breakdown of what your eating schedule might look like:

- 1st meal of the day: noon
- 2nd meal of the day: 4:00 p.m.
- 3rd meal of the day: 8:00 p.m.

Or

- 1st meal of the day: 1:00 p.m.
- 2nd meal of the day: 5:00 p.m.
- 3rd meal of the day: 9:00 p.m.

The main point is that you want to fast for 16 hours a day, and then have a feeding window of 8 hours. You can start and end your fasts at whatever time you like as long as you're skipping breakfast and not eating for a couple of hours before going to bed.

Also, you don't have to space out each meal equally apart from each other. For example, if eating your second meal of the day at 4:00 is too early, then you could eat your first meal at noon and your second meal at 5:00 when you get off of work.

Then you could eat your third meal at 8:00 or even at a different time. While this is my favorite method of fasting, it's not the only way that you can go about doing things.

There could be special circumstances where you're not going to be able to fast for 14-16 hours in the day. For example, you might be on vacation, and your eating schedule might get thrown out of whack because you're not in control as much for when you're eating.

What should you do in cases like these? You should delay eating your first meal of the day for as long as possible, preferably for at least 5 hours.

For example, if you wake up at 10:00 a.m., then fast for as long as possible after you wake up. Ideally, you'd fast for at least 5 hours until 3:00 p.m.

Since you're on vacation, that might not be possible; if that's the case, simply fast for as long as you can after you wake up. If that means your first meal is at 1:00 and you only fasted for 3 hours after waking, then great.

Yes, this means you're going to have to skip the hotel breakfast, but it'll be worth it. You don't want to use your vacation as an excuse to eat however you please.

You still want to have some sort of plan in place. This way, you'll get the best of both worlds.

You'll still have a fasting plan in place, while at the same time be able to enjoy yourself if you're staying up later than usual eating and drinking. Remember though, this is for special circumstances only.

Most of the time, you're going to aim to fast for 14-16 hours per day and then eat within the 8-hour feeding window. Finally, be sure to check out the frequently asked questions chapter where I cover some common questions about fasting in more depth.

Step 5: Implement and Adjust as Necessary

You now have the foundation you need in order to start your diet plan. What you need to do is finish the rest of this book and then get started as soon as possible.

Nothing will help you learn faster along the way than experience. Start tracking all of your calories and macros.

At first, this won't be the easiest thing to do. However, as time goes on, you'll get better and better at it.

Don't give up on it if it takes a bit of time to get used to. You'll also need to weigh yourself to see if you're making progress or not.

Sadly, most people go about doing this in the wrong way. For instance, they might weigh themselves every day or at different times of the day.

The problem with weighing yourself every day is that our bodyweight fluctuates. The number on the scale is influenced by things such as food in the stomach, or how hydrated you are.

Therefore, if you're weighing yourself every day, you're not getting an accurate measure of if you're truly losing fat or not. Your bodyweight could fluctuate upwards one day and down the next.

Not only that, but imagine what this will do to your psyche. You might step on the scale one day, excited to see that you've lost half a pound.

Then the next day you step on the scale and get disappointed because it shows that you gained a pound. The reality is that you didn't actually gain a pound overnight, your bodyweight is simply fluctuating.

That's why the best thing you can do when it comes to weighing yourself is to weigh yourself periodically enough to account for fluctuations. When you step on the scale, you need to feel confident that it's an accurate reading as to whether you've gained or lost weight.

Weighing yourself once a week will let you know if you're heading in the right direction or not.

In addition, you need to make sure that you weigh yourself at the same time every single time you step on the scale. If you weigh yourself upon waking up one week and in the middle of the afternoon the next, then the reading won't be as consistent.

The best practice is to weigh yourself soon after waking up, right after you go to the bathroom. This way you're weighing yourself on an empty stomach with similar hydration levels every single time.

After tracking your bodyweight for a couple of weeks, you'll want to see if you're making progress or not. If you're losing one pound per week, then great, keep on doing what you're doing.

If you're not losing any weight, or if you're possibly gaining weight, then you need to take a step back and evaluate the situation. The first thing you need to make sure of is that you're accurately tracking your calories and macros.

This is usually where mistakes happen, which can cause you to not get any results. Inaccuracies can happen sometimes because you're not used to correctly measuring portion sizes, and it can take some practice to get good at that.

Other times though, people will feel ashamed to log certain foods that they're eating, or they might cheat and put in smaller portion sizes than they're eating. Remember that no one is going to see your food log expect for you.

You don't have to worry about being judged by anyone. At the end of the day, if you're not doing your best to accurately log what you're eating, then you're only cheating yourself.

This is for your own benefit, so you might as well do it.

The cool thing about tracking all of your calories is that you can see what you've eaten over the past few weeks as well. Look at your food log and see if you notice any commonalities that may have caused you to overeat.

Did you eat too much fast food? Do you eat and drink too much when you're going out with your friends?

By tracking and logging your food intake, patterns will start to appear. Look at certain high-calorie food items that could be holding you back and eat less of them.

See if you've been able to stick to a 14-16 hour fast daily. Are you drinking too much soda or other beverages that contain a high amount of calories?

If so, then these are some areas that you can improve on. The final thing you'll want to consider is if you're adding muscle while dropping fat at the same time.

For example, the number on the scale might not be changing much, and that could be due to the fact that you're replacing the fat you're burning with muscle. If you're lifting weights and want to build muscle, then this isn't a bad thing by any means.

It is something you'll want to be aware of though; you might think that you're not making any progress when, in reality, you are. The last thing you would want to do in a scenario like this is make changes to your diet plan when you don't need to.

If you feel you're adding muscle too quickly, then you could scale back on the weightlifting routine some. Diet wise though, you're doing everything you need to in order to head towards your goals.

Of course, if you think this may be happening to you, then you'll need a way to measure your body fat percentage to make sure that you're heading in the right direction.

As long as your body fat percentage is going down, then you're doing the right thing. The trick is to make sure that you're getting a proper measurement.

One common way people measure their body fat is by using skinfold calipers. These tend to be inaccurate because most people don't have much experience using them.

You have to use the caliper in the same spots in the same exact way for the best accuracy and most people mess it up. If you're going to use skinfold calipers to measure your body fat, make sure you see a professional who has plenty of experience using them.

The best way to get your body fat percentage measured is to use something known as a DEXA scan. This is considered the gold standard for body fat testing in the fitness world.

You'll simply lie down and let the machine scan over you for a couple of minutes. Not only will this tell you what your body fat percentage is, but it'll also measure your muscle mass as well as your bone mass.

The only problem with it is the price. It can cost upwards of 100 dollars or more depending on your location.

Also, it might not be that convenient for you to make appointments to get your body fat tested. This is however, extremely accurate.

If you wanted to, you could get a DEXA scan done at the start of your fitness journey and later on once you've made some considerable progress. If you want a much cheaper option that's easier to use than calipers and can be done in the comfort of your own home, then bioelectrical impedance could be for you.

You can buy it as a handheld device, and it even comes as a feature on some weight scales. It works by sending a small electrical current through your body.

The amount of time it takes for the current to pass through your body will determine what your body fat percentage is. Accuracy wise, this method certainly isn't as good as a DEXA scan.

The readings can vary quite a bit depending on things such as your hydration level, or if you've recently consumed a meal. Dehydration for example, can increase electrical resistance and cause a higher body fat reading.

However, the thing we care about here is consistency. If you're going to use bioelectrical impedance as a way to measure your body fat, then keep things the same every time you use it.

The best way to go about this would be to take your measurement soon after waking up. Similar to how you would weigh yourself first thing in the morning, you could take your body fat reading as well.

Yes, you'll be dehydrated in the morning which will affect the result, but at least you'll have similar levels of dehydration every time you use the device. If on the other hand, you measure your body fat at random times of the day, you might be more hydrated one day than another.

Or the meal you just ate may affect the reading. It may not be the most accurate way to measure your body fat, but it should be able to give you an idea if you're heading in the right direction or not.

And due to the inaccuracies of common ways to measure your body fat, I recommend you only consider regularly measuring your body fat in special circumstances. Namely, this would be if you think you're losing fat and gaining muscle at the same time, causing your overall weight to stay the same.

The weight reading on the scale is going to be the best way to go about things in terms of cost, ease of use, and accuracy, assuming you're weighing yourself in a consistent manner every time.

Also, don't forget that the main thing you want to be concerned with is how you look in the mirror. If you're noticing results with how you look in the mirror, then you know you're on the right track.

However, sometimes it can take a bit of time before you notice significant changes in the way that you look. That's why you want to make sure you have a way of measuring your progress along the way, which is going to be a weight scale in the majority of cases.

Now that we've covered the basic steps you need to take to get your diet plan up and running, let's get into specifics on what you should eat...

What Should I Eat on This Endomorph Diet Plan?

As I've talked about before, the big problem with a lot of mainstream diets is that they tell you what you can and can't eat. One diet might say that you can never eat anything with sugar in it ever again.

Yes, I agree that not eating sugar is a very healthy thing to do. However, is it realistic to think that someone could go the rest of his or her life without consuming sugar ever again?

Sure there's going to be that rare case, but it's few and far between. Most people would fail on such a diet plan because we are biologically hardwired to seek out sugary and salty foods due to their richness in calories.

No, this isn't an excuse to eat these types of foods all of the time. Instead, it's wiser to limit sugar intake, but not get rid of it altogether.

This way you'll still be able to enjoy your favorite foods that contain sugar from time to time, such as brownies or cake. And it's because of unsustainable diet plans such as no sugar diets that cause people to get caught in the vicious yo-yo dieting cycle.

They'll put themselves through misery to lose weight, only to quit when they can't take it anymore and then slowly start to gain all of the weight back. That's why I'm not going to tell you specifically what you can and cannot eat.

I want this to be a long-term approach where you're able to lose weight and keep it off for good. That's why I'm instead going to give you guidelines for what kinds of foods you should eat, and then you can fill in the rest.

If I told you what to eat for every single meal, that would be like you riding a bike using training wheels. The training wheels are the only thing that allow you to be able to successfully ride the bike.

What would happen if you were in a situation where you couldn't eat what I told you to? The training wheels would be taken away and you'd struggle to ride the bike.

This approach will make you much better off for long-term success because you'll be more in tune with your own body.

Follow My Golden 85% Rule

When it comes to eating your favorite foods versus healthy foods, how do you go about striking a balance? Eating junk food all of the time will make it extremely difficult to keep your overall calories low.

Not only that, but you'll be dealing with a lot of food cravings thanks to the blood sugar crashes. Eating healthy all of the time can lead to burnout, causing you to binge eat and feel guilty about yourself.

That's why you should eat healthy foods 85% of the time and the remaining 15% of the time eat foods you enjoy. This allows you to strike the perfect balance between clean foods and junk food.

Remember it's not what you eat 15% of the time that causes obesity problems—it's what you eat the majority of the time that causes problems. What exactly constitutes something as healthy though?

My general rule is to think of our ancestors. If it wasn't possible for them to eat something back in the day, then it should be part of the 15%.

You want to consume foods that contain as few of ingredients as possible. Now, this isn't a hard and fast rule.

For example, let's say you're going to have pasta for dinner one night. If you're worried about whether or not white pasta should go in the 15% category, then you're overthinking things.

Put it in the 85% and move on. Generally, you know what's good and what's not.

Sugary desserts and salty snacks like potato chips go in the 15% category. These are foods that you want to enjoy from time to time.

Things like vegetables and lean meats should go into the 85% category. Here's a non-comprehensive list of some healthy foods you could eat as part of your diet plan:

- Fruits
- Vegetables
- Sweet potatoes
- Brown Rice
- Avocados
- Various types of nuts and seeds
- Different kinds of beans
- Quinoa
- Cottage cheese
- Coconut oil

You might also be wondering how you know if you're eating a proper ratio of healthy to unhealthy foods. Well just like with the macros, it's doesn't have to be spot on.

Just try to get around those numbers. Over the course of a week, it should average out to roughly 85% healthy foods and 15% not so healthy foods.

You can take these percentages and factor them into your total caloric intake. For example, if I'm eating 2,230 calories per day, then approximately 335 of those calories can come from junk food.

The remaining 1,895 should come from clean sources. In this example, 335 calories per day might not seem like a lot, but remember you can divide it up how you like.

You could eat all 335 calories every single day, which would maybe mean eating a small bowl of ice cream or some potato chips. Or you could save up those calories and use them for later.

For instance, you could go three days eating only healthy foods, which would allow you to eat a meal consisting of 1,005 calories of whatever you wanted. Finally, you could even save up all of your junk calories for one day of the week where you can essentially have a cheat day.

The choice is yours. You do want to make sure that you're still properly counting and tracking your macros.

To be clear, these aren't extra calories that you're adding into your diet plan. You're still going to eat the same amount of calories and macros that we calculated earlier.

Let's say for instance you eat some candy that contains 30 grams of carbs. You still need to factor that in towards your 25% total daily carbohydrates that you're going to be eating for the day.

Chapter 4: Why Me? The Correct Endomorph Mindset You Need to Have

Having the correct mindset is something that most people struggle with when it comes to achieving their health and fitness goals. However, as an endomorph, it's especially critical that you have the proper mindset to ensure success with your health and fitness goals.

The main reason for this is because it can be easy to compare yourself to people who are naturally slender, and wonder why you couldn't have been born with a metabolism like theirs. This mindset is what can then hold you back from taking the action necessary in order to reach your goals.

If you don't think that diet or exercise will work for you, then you won't take the necessary action and you'll stay stuck.

That's why it's so important to make sure you have the proper mentality to realize that it is possible for you to be able to achieve your goals, regardless of how many times you've failed in the past, or if you've been overweight your whole life. None of that matters.

All that matters is the present moment and where you're going from this day forward. That's the first thing I need you to do—let go of anything from your past that might be holding you back.

Forgive yourself and move forward. You owe it to your future self. I know how bad it can be to hold onto failures from the past.

For instance, I have many regrets from my senior season of high school basketball. My team didn't achieve the goals that I had in mind for the season, and as the leader of the team, I felt like I let a lot of people down—especially myself.

In fact, I still have dreams about my senior season to this very day. I'm telling you from my own personal experience that you have to let the past be the past, even if it's really hard.

You have to use it as a learning experience. For instance, this whole experience has taught me that I have to do everything in my power to achieve a certain outcome that I want.

I can't leave anything on the table because if I do, then I might end up with the same regret that I did back when I was in high school. The best way that I've been able to help myself move on from this was to forgive myself.

I didn't have all the knowledge back then that I have now. In fact, I wouldn't be where I am today if it weren't for my past failures and mistakes.

I'm sure the same can be said for you. Maybe you've tried dieting and exercising in the past and it didn't work for you.

It's okay if that's the case. Simply forgive yourself because you probably didn't have the right information.

Back then, you didn't know everything that you're learning in this book. So use your past failures as learning experiences.

At least now you know some things that didn't work for you. That's great!

You don't have to worry about wasting your time on those things in the future. Forgiveness and permission to be imperfect are the best ways to move on from the past.

The reality is that even with the right information, there will still be times when you slip up or make mistakes, which leads me to my next tip...

How You Should Handle Setbacks

Even if you have moved on from the past, the reality is that mistakes you make in the present can trip you up too. These mistakes will then become a recent memory in your past, which can then hold you back in the future.

That's why when a mistake does happen and you fall down, you must get back up immediately and keep on moving forward as if nothing happened. That's the best way to handle setbacks.

The more you sit there and dwell and worry about your mistake, the more it'll keep popping up in your mind to try and sabotage you. You have to remember that work beats worry.

If you get right back up and keep on working towards your goal, that depressing thought will lose its power and go away. It's easy to see how mistakes made along the way could trip up even the most enthusiastic of individuals.

You make a mistake, and then you start to wonder why you did that. Then thinking of that thought makes you think about it even more.

Then the mistake will start to paralyze you from taking any action in the future. And once the action stops, so do the results that you're getting.

Therefore, the best thing you can do is always be laser-focused on moving forward. Get that tunnel vision and move forward at all costs.

Another thing you can do to help yourself with this is to remind yourself that you're imperfect. If you try to be perfect and then fail, your mind won't hesitate to let you know that you did an action that's inconsistent with the perfect person you're supposed to be.

However, if you embrace your imperfections instead, then you're essentially telling yourself that you're human and you make mistakes from time to time. Then when a mistake does happen, it's not the end of the world.

You'll find that it will be much easier to move on from it.

Why You Shouldn't Compare Yourself to Others

A point I briefly mentioned earlier is that you shouldn't compare yourself to others. Doing so will only make you feel worse about yourself and wonder why it is that you have to go through the struggles that you do while others don't.

Playing the comparison game is one that you'll never be able to win. So if you regularly notice that you compare yourself to others, what are some things that you can do?

The first thing I want you to take a look at is your social media use. There is research to show that there is a correlation between social media usage and depression (2). That is to say that the more time you spend on social media, the more likely it is that you're going to have some degree of depression.

Why is that? Well think about what it is that you see when you log onto any of the popular social media sites—you see all sorts of amazing and exciting things!

This person bought a new house, so and so got a new promotion, a friend from high school just got engaged, somebody had a kid, somebody else just had a killer workout and on and on it goes. Social media is a highlight of people's lives.

And that makes total sense. People are only going to share the best and most exciting things that are happening in their lives in order to generate the most likes.

And when you constantly see these things, it's going to make you feel like you're not adequate. You're going to wonder why you're struggling to get fit while everyone else is living their dream life with fulfilling work, relationships, and travel to cool places.

The reality is that a lot of social media is an exaggerated truth. People will make their lives seem better than they actually are in order to get more attention on social media.

The game of seeing what posts or pictures can generate the most likes is a never-ending cycle. The fact of the matter is that a lot of our lives consist of boring and mundane things—driving to work, eating, sleeping, watching t.v., etc.

Rarely do exciting things happen. Yet when you're friends with 500 people on social media, it can sure make it seem as if something new and exciting is happening all of the time.

Guess what though? It's not!

That's why the best thing you can do is limit or eliminate entirely the use of social media. This will help you not compare yourself to others as much.

I noticed big leaps in my happiness once I stopped using social media. Of course, if you want to use it to connect with an old friend and actually meet up to hang out with him or her in person, then go for it.

For the most part though, you're definitely better off not using it and instead focusing on what it is that you need to do in order to reach your goals.

If you're able to limit or stop using social media altogether, then congratulations! You've taken a major step towards not comparing yourself to others. You won't know how good it'll be for you until you try, so definitely give it a shot!

However, that's not the only thing that you need to do. There's still a lot of other stimulation we receive every day from advertisements.

These ads are designed to make us want to desire a certain thing. It might be a "flawless" model trying to sell us makeup for example.

And if only we had this thing, then it would finally be the key we need to unlock our happiness. Of course, that's rarely the case.

Therefore you also need to limit the stimulation you receive from ads. This isn't the easiest thing to do.

No matter what, you're not going to be able to stop seeing all ads unless you decide to live under a rock. Even with that being the case, there are still some practical things you can do to help limit the use of ad stimulation.

You might be wondering how all of this ties into losing weight as an endomorph, but trust me, all of these things affect our mindset and our moods, which in turn determines our actions, which determines our results. Mindset really could be the thing that's been holding you back, so please give this advice a shot before you immediately dismiss it.

Number #1: Limit use of the radio

When you're driving your car to work, the grocery store, or wherever else, I want you to consider doing something besides listening to the radio. The reason for this is not just to avoid the ads, but also because of the songs that you'll be listening to.

What are most songs today about? Usually, it's about love or getting money depending on the genre of the song.

And if you're single or broke, this can really make you feel depressed. You might think that the reason why you're single is that you're struggling to get fit.

I'm not saying that you should never listen to the radio or music in general ever again. What I want you to do is to start paying attention to how you feel after listening to mainstream music on the radio.

Then give up the radio for a couple of weeks and see how you feel. Notice how you feel after listening to certain genres, maybe you need to listen to different kinds of music.

The reality is that music can negatively or positively affect our moods and our thoughts—as some research indicates (3). Therefore you need to be more conscious of the kind of music that you do listen to in order to ensure that music isn't subconsciously affecting your mood in a negative way.

And finally, if you're not sure of what else to do in your car if you're not going to listen to music, then consider listening to podcasts, audiobooks, or just have complete silence. There's nothing wrong with some quiet time every now and then!

Number #2: Be smart about watching television

The next big way most of us see ads is during breaks on the television shows we watch. Again the more ads we're exposed to, the more likely it is to negatively affect our mindset and thus our ability to get results.

Therefore it's wise to limit the use of, if not stop watching t.v. altogether. You may not want to stop watching t.v. altogether and if so that's okay.

But you do need to be more conscious about how you're consuming it. For instance, you could pre-record your shows and then watch them later.

This will allow you to be able to fast forward through the ads when they come on. You could also watch your shows using an online subscription service that doesn't contain any ads.

Number #3: Use an ad blocker when you're on the internet

The final thing you can do to limit the number of ads that you see is to use an ad blocker on your internet browser. This will block ads that you'd normally see when you're browsing through articles on the internet.

Again every little bit helps, so try this out and see what kind of a difference it makes.

The Correct Way to Set Goals to Increase Your Chances of Success

Most of the world doesn't set goals. Most people don't really know what it is that they want, or they have a vague idea of what they want to achieve.

Imagine being an archer but not having a target to aim and shoot at. It's impossible to win!

On the contrary, imagine having a laser focus on the target you're trying to shoot. Nothing else is distracting you from hitting the bull's eye.

By setting goals, you'll be able to focus in on what it is that you truly want. Things won't be able to easily distract you anymore.

Setting goals will make what you want real; if used right, they'll also create a sense of urgency that will encourage you to take the necessary action in order to accomplish your goals. Here's the wrong way to go about setting a goal:

- I want to lose weight.

This is nothing more than a vague idea in your head. If it happens then great, but no big deal if it doesn't.

It's as if your goal is in a bottle in the middle of the ocean and you're hoping it'll magically find its way to the correct destination. Here's a much more powerful way to set your goals:

- I lose 10 pounds of fat by January 31, 2019.

So what is it that makes writing your goals in this manner so much more effective? Well, the first thing is that you need to write it down physically with pen and paper.

This makes your goal real and not an idea in your head. Ideally, you would write your goal down first thing in the morning and before you go to bed each night.

This way it'll be what you think about when you first wake up and the last thing you think about before you go to bed. Secondly, the goal is written in the present tense as if it's already been achieved.

This has a much more powerful effect on the subconscious than saying something like 'I will lose 10 pounds of fat'. The reason is that it makes your mind think that you've already achieved the goal.

Your subconscious mind doesn't know the difference between something that's real versus something that's being vividly imagined. Therefore, we can take advantage of this by acting as if we've already achieved our goal, and imagining what it would look and feel like to have accomplished this goal.

This goal is also specific. It targets a certain amount of weight to be lost.

Instead of generally saying you want to lose weight, you have a specific number in mind. Not only that, but what kind of weight do you want to lose? Muscle mass? Water weight?

I'm assuming what you want to lose is fat. That's why the goal says to lose 10 pounds of *fat*.

This gives us a specific target to aim for. The final thing you'll notice about this goal is that there's a deadline attached to it.

If you don't put a deadline to your goals, then it's as if you're saying to yourself, "I'll get around to achieving this when I have the extra time." And you and I know good and well that time will likely never come.

That's why you must set a deadline for when you'll achieve your goal. Remember there's no such thing as an unrealistic goal, just unrealistic time frames.

If your deadline ends up being too ambitious and you don't reach your goal by then, don't sweat it. You can always set a new deadline for when you'll achieve the goal by.

The main thing is that you don't skip this creating a deadline. A deadline will help create the urgency necessary in order for you to be able to get the job done in a timely manner.

Find Your Why

After you set a goal for what it is that you want to achieve, the next thing that you need to do is find your why. Finding your why is a powerful motivator that can help drive you to achieve your goal.

Similar with setting goals, there's a right and a wrong way to go about doing this. If you have an idea as to why you want to achieve something in your head, that likely isn't strong enough for you to be able to get the job done.

Just like with writing your goals down, you also need to write your reason why down. Not only that, most people only scratch the surface when it comes to finding their why.

Someone might say for example that he or she wants to get healthy. However, that might only be a surface reason for what the person truly wants.

You must dive deeper. The best way to do that is to ask yourself why three times. For example:

Why do you want to lose weight?

I want to look and feel better about myself.

Why do you want to look and feel better about yourself?

So I can go out on more dates.

Why do you want to go out on more dates?

So I can be in a relationship.

Therefore, the main thing that would be driving this person would be so that he or she can be in a relationship. If he or she stopped with "I want to look and feel better about myself", then he or she likely wouldn't be motivated to keep on moving forward.

That reason wouldn't be compelling enough. However, now that we got to the root of what it is that the person truly wants, this can be a much more powerful motivator.

At the end of the day, we're all driven by something, so you might as well find out what it is that you truly want and then go for it. Think about it in this way—why do some people stick around at a job they hate for years on end?

Asking why can help us get to the bottom of that:

Why do I work at a job that I loathe?

So I can pay for my bills.

Why do I want to pay my bills?

So I can afford to eat and have a roof over my head.

Why do I want to eat and have a roof over my head?

Because starving and not having a place to live would be worse than going back to my job.

So in the end, staying at a job someone hates is easier and better than not being able to eat or have a place to live. Staying at a job you hate can also be easier than updating your resume, applying for a new job, interviewing, hoping you get the job, and then learning the ins and outs of the new job.

When you think of all that you have to do in order to get a new job, it can be much easier to stay put where you're at. That's why, when it comes to weight loss or any other endeavor worth achieving, you must focus on the next step and nothing else.

For example, when you think about all that you have to do in order to workout at the gym—change into workout clothes, drive to the gym, workout, come home, and shower, it can be quite daunting.

However, if you only think about the next step, then things won't seem as bad. If you told yourself all I'm going to do is change into gym clothes, then that's a lot less intimidating than the thought of everything else you'll have to do.

Then once your gym clothes are on, ask yourself what the next step is and do that. Before you know it, you'll have completed the entire process of going to the gym without it feeling like such a big chore.

To think of it in another way, imagine your life like an hourglass. In an hourglass, only one grain of sand can pass through at a time. Yes, sand is continuously passing through the hourglass, but it still is coming through one grain at a time.

Much is the same in our lives. Time is continually passing us by regardless of what we do.

Even with that being the case, there's still only one thing we can do before we move onto the next thing. For example, you don't change your clothes and appear at the gym to workout all at once.

You change your clothes, then you drive to the gym, and then you workout. Breaking your tasks up into smaller chunks makes it far easier to consume and makes it more likely that you'll actually do it.

And speaking of things you need to do in order to achieve your goals, let's not forget about process goals...

Don't Forget About Process Goals

There are outcome goals and process goals. The type of goal we talked about earlier is an outcome goal.

Process goals are what you have to do in order to achieve your outcome goals. It helps if you think of this as a mountain—the outcome goal is like the top of a mountain; it's where you want to go.

Process goals are what you must do in order to reach the top of the mountain. Here's an example:

Outcome goal: I lose 10 pounds of fat by January 31, 2019.

Process goal: I workout 3 days per week at 7:00 a.m. Monday, Wednesday, and Friday.

Having a desired outcome is great, but that won't do you much good if you don't have a game plan laid out for what it is that you need to do in order to achieve that outcome goal.

And when I'm talking about a plan, I'm talking about a specific one. Notice how the process goal wasn't something vague like, "I workout 3 days per week."

It needs to be more specific than that. What time are you going to workout at? What days of the week, etc.?

Make sure you have a plan in place for each process goal. This will make it all the more likely that you'll actually do what you need to do.

Remember that failing to prepare is setting yourself up for failure, and having vague process goals is telling yourself that it's not that important.

The final question then becomes, how many process goals should you have? Working out 3 days per week is great, but that may not be the only thing you need to do in order to reach your goal.

That's why I recommend that you have 3 process goals with every one outcome goal that you have. Think to yourself about what the 3 main things are that you need to do in order to be successful.

In the case of losing 10 pounds of fat, it could be something like:

1. Exercising a certain amount.
2. Eating a certain number of meals that consist of healthy food choices.
3. Getting the proper amount of sleep.

Of course, saying you'll get the proper amount of sleep or making healthy food choices isn't specific enough. Everyone knows that they need to do that, and yet most people struggle to do these things on a regular basis.

Here's a better way to make them more specific:

- I eat three meals per day at noon, 4:00 p.m. and 8:00 p.m. My meals consist of wholesome food choices that are high in protein, moderate in fat, and low in carbs.
- I sleep for 8 hours each and every night. I go to bed at 11:00 p.m. and wake up at 7:00 a.m. 7 days per week.

Hopefully, you can notice a difference in making your process goals specific.

Now you have a much better game plan moving forward as to what it is you need to do in order to achieve your outcome goal.

Are you enjoying this book so far? If so, please consider leaving a review. Even just a few words would help others decide if the book is right for them!

Chapter 5: Endomorph Exercise—How to Workout in a Way That's Optimal for Your Body Type

Make no mistake about it—you don't *have* to exercise in order to achieve your weight loss goals. However, it'll make things much easier on yourself, especially as an endomorph.

Think of exercise as a bonus; it'll either give you some more leeway in your nutrition plan, or it'll help you reach your goal that much faster. The reason why I say that you don't have to exercise in order to get results is that you can lose weight by focusing solely on your nutrition plan.

If your diet plan is solid, then that alone could be enough to get you to where you want to go. The reality is that you can't out-exercise a bad diet.

So for example, you could eat a burger, fries, and milkshake at a fast food restaurant. That meal could easily contain at least 2,000 calories.

Needless to say, it would take a very very long time in order for you to burn off the equivalent to that. You would almost have to run the equivalent of a marathon in order to fully burn off that meal.

That's not a fair deal. The better way to go about things is to not eat that meal in the first place.

That way any exercise you do can be seen as a bonus instead of a desperate attempt to make up for something you shouldn't have eaten.

What Kind of Exercise Should You Do?

One of the characteristics of an endomorph is that they're the strongest and contain the most muscle mass of the 3 different body types. With that being the case, it makes sense to do exercise routines that are based on those strengths.

Doing something like long and boring cardio probably isn't the best option for endomorphs. It's a common myth that doing cardio is the best way to burn fat.

The reality is that exercise burns calories, and burning calories will help to put you into a caloric deficit, which is how your body will burn fat. Therefore, you shouldn't worry as much about the type of exercise that you're doing.

Instead, focus on what your strengths are and what you enjoy doing. That's what you'll stick to in the long run.

It doesn't matter how good an exercise plan is, if you quit and give up on it, then it won't work. That's why I want you to do something that's more fun than jogging on a treadmill.

Not only that, but you might as well exercise in a way that's optimal for your body type. So what type of exercise should you do?

Well if you shouldn't do slow cardio, then you should do the opposite. The opposite of slow is high intensity and the opposite of running is resistance training.

Therefore the type of exercise that's best for an endomorph is high-intensity resistance training.

Why High-Intensity Workouts are Best for Endomorphs

So what is it exactly that makes high-intensity workouts so great for endomorphs? Well consider this—endomorphs have the slowest metabolisms of the 3 different body types.

Therefore, endomorphs need to do workouts that will help to increase their metabolisms. You're definitely not going to have that happen by doing slow cardio.

However, if you lift as heavy as possible and keep the rest periods short, this will keep your heart rate up, and as a result, help to boost your metabolism. Not only that, but an endomorph's body was designed to workout in this type of manner.

It was made to do high-intensity work for short periods of time. An ectomorph was made to do something more along the lines of long-distance work such as a marathon.

You'll probably enjoy doing these types of workouts more than going on a 5-mile run for example.

Endomorph Workout

The ideal endomorph workout is one where you're first and foremost training with mostly compound exercises. A compound exercise is one that works on multiple muscle groups at the same time.

An example of this would be the barbell squat. The squat primarily works on the quads, hamstrings, and glutes.

On the other hand, an isolation exercise primarily works on one muscle group at a time. An example of an isolation exercise is something like a leg extension.

The leg extension only works on the quads. Filling your workout routine with a bunch of isolation exercises would be a waste of your time in the sense that you won't be doing things as efficiently and effectively as you could be.

After that, you want to make sure that you're training with higher rep ranges—around 12-15 reps per set. A rep is a single completion of an exercise.

On the squat for example, you would squat down and then stand back up. That would be one rep of the exercise.

A set is a series of reps. For example, if you were doing 3 sets of 12 reps on squat, you would squat down and then come back up completing one rep of the exercise.

You would do that 11 more times and that would complete 1 set of the exercise. You would then take a rest period (in this case let's say one minute) and once the rest period is over you would complete another 12 reps for set number 2, rest again for one minute and then complete set number 3 by doing another 12 reps.

Once all 3 sets of 12 reps have been completed, you would then move onto the next exercise in the workout routine. The reason why we want to do higher reps here is that this is going to help to keep the heart rate up.

It'll help to keep the intensity of the workout high and allow you to burn more calories overall. Don't get me wrong, training in lower rep ranges and taking longer rest periods certainly has its place, especially if you're a powerlifter or something along those lines.

However, for the average endomorph who's looking to optimize his or her time in the gym to maximize fat-burn, this is going to be the best way to go about doing things. Speaking of rest periods, you'll want to rest for 30-60 seconds in between sets for your exercises.

This again will help to keep your heart rate up and make sure that the workout stays intense. If you take 3-5 minutes of rest in between sets, then that's enough time for your heart rate to come down some.

The final thing you need to consider is how heavy of a weight you should use. A good rule to follow is that you always want to lift as heavy of a weight as possible for the given rep range.

So if you were completing 5 reps of an exercise, you're going to use more weight than if you were doing 15 reps for the same exercise. However, that doesn't mean you should use so light of a weight that the 15 reps isn't challenging.

You want the last 1-2 reps of the exercise to be extremely challenging. In fact, it's better to pick a weight that's too heavy and causes you to fail at rep number 13 out of 15 than it is to pick a weight that's too light and stop at 15 when you could've done more.

It comes down to having the right mentality. If the workout says to get 15 reps and we're not sure how much weight to use, we tend to err on the side of a weight that's too light.

Even though we could push ourselves past 15 reps, we stop at 15 because that's what our workout told us to do. You might not know how much weight you should be using if it's your first time doing an exercise, so at that point take your best guess.

If you're able to easily get 15 reps without any sort of challenge, then increase the weight for the next set. Keep adjusting the weight as necessary until you get to the point where the last 1-2 reps are very challenging.

And over time, you want to make sure that you're increasing the amount of weight that you're lifting. If you lift the same weight with the same exercises and the same reps, your body will catch on to what you're doing and progress will stall.

Therefore, whenever you can successfully complete all of the reps for a given exercise, increase the weight the next time you do the exercise. Let's use an example of doing 3 sets of 15 reps of the dumbbell military press exercise:

Workout #1: Weight being used — 30-pound dumbbells

- Set 1:15 reps
- Set 2:13 reps
- Set 3: 12 reps

Since the lifter wasn't able to complete 15 reps on sets 2 and 3 he should stick with the 30-pound dumbbells until he can do 15 reps on all 3 sets. Let's say on his next workout he is able to complete 15 reps on all 3 sets using the 30-pound dumbbells.

That's great, and for the next workout he should increase the weight to the next set of heavier dumbbells. In most gyms, this will likely mean using 35-pound dumbbells.

And if on his first time using 35-pound dumbbells he's unable to hit 15 reps per set that's okay. He'll stick with that same weight until he's able to do 15 reps for all 3 sets and then increase the weight once again.

This is a principle known as progressive overload, which states that you always need to be challenging your body in order for it to keep on growing. That's why with each and every workout you want to try and increase the number of reps you're doing or the amount of weight that you lift.

For example, let's say that you're aiming to complete 12 reps of an exercise. The first time you do it, you get 12 reps on the first set, 11 on the second, and 9 on the third set.

The next time you do that exercise, strive to do more reps on your second and third sets. You still might not hit 12 reps on all 3 sets, but maybe you'll be able to do 12 on the first, 12 on the second, and 11 on the third.

That's great because you're still making process and giving your body a challenge. You would still stick with that weight until you're able to do 12 reps on all 3 sets before increasing the weight.

Here's a sample full body workout that you can do in the gym 2-3 days per week:

- Dumbbell Squats: 3 sets of 12 reps, 60 seconds rest between sets
- Dumbbell Bench Press: 3 sets of 12 reps, 60 seconds rest between sets
- Lat Pulldowns: 3 sets of 12 reps, 60 seconds rest between sets
- Standing Dumbbell Military Press: 3 sets of 15 reps, 45 seconds rest between sets
- Standing Dumbbell Curls: 3 sets of 15 reps, 30 seconds rest between sets
- Tricep Pushdowns: 3 sets of 15 reps, 30 seconds rest between sets

Don't let the simplicity of this workout fool you. Often times it's the simplest things that are the most effective.

Doing this workout 2-3 times per week will give you some great benefits. Many people sadly think that full body workouts are a waste of time and instead prefer a bro-splits routine, where you only workout one muscle group per session.

Full body workouts are going to be awesome for you as an endomorph for the following reasons:

- You'll burn more calories in less time thanks to the metabolically demanding compound exercises.
- You'll experience a better recovery of your nervous system because you won't be lifting weights on consecutive days.
- You'll be able to gain strength and build muscle faster since you're working out your major muscle groups multiple times per week.
- And if you're new to weight training, you'll master the exercises sooner because you'll be performing them more often.

Make sure you have at least one day of rest in between each workout. For example, if you're working out 3 days per week you could workout on a Monday, Wednesday, and Friday.

Should I Not Waste My Time Doing Cardio as an Endomorph?

It's not that you shouldn't do any cardio as an endomorph. Cardio can still give you some good results if you do it in the right way.

Doing cardio in the wrong way is a waste of your time because you're not doing things as efficiently as you could be. That's why I want to share with you the most effective way to do cardio.

The reason why I say this is because it allows you to burn the most amount of calories in the least amount of time. Here's the first part of the cardio workout:

High-intensity interval training

High-intensity interval training (HIIT for short) is essentially where you alternate between a period of high-intensity exercise and a period of low-intensity exercise. For example, if you were doing a HIIT workout on a treadmill, you might alternate between running at a speed of 7mph and walking at a speed of 3 mph.

This is way better than doing something like jogging. The reason is that this type of intense workout fits perfectly with the endomorph body type.

HIIT will do a better job of helping you reach your max heart rate. It'll do a better job of boosting your metabolism compared to slow and steady state cardio.

Now you can do HIIT on any cardio machine of your choice whether that be that a treadmill, an elliptical, a stairmaster, a rowing machine, or even on an outdoor track. Whatever you choose doesn't matter.

What does matter is that you alternate between a high-intensity and a low-intensity. Let's say for example, you're doing your HIIT workout on a treadmill.

How fast should you run for during the high-intensity part and at what pace should you go for the low-intensity part? Basically, for the high-intensity part of the workout, I recommend going at a pace where you would be pushing yourself.

Not so much to the point where you might pass out, but to where it's a challenge. That will be different speeds for different people.

For some people that might mean running at 10 mph, for others 7 mph, or maybe 6 mph. Your high-intensity speed will also depend on the duration of the intense exercise.

For example, there are many different high-intensity to low-intensity ratios you can do. You could run for a minute and walk for a minute.

You could do 30 seconds of running and 1 minute of walking. You might also do 1 minute of running and 2 minutes of walking.

The point is to adjust things based on your current fitness level. Ideally, you'd work your way up to a 1:1 ratio where you're running for the same length of time that you're walking.

Initially though, you might not be at that point. And thanks to the efficiency of this workout, you can burn quite a few calories in a short period of time such as 15 minutes. Here's an example HIIT workout you could do on a treadmill:

High-Intensity Exercise for 30 seconds consisting of running on a treadmill at 7 mph.

Alternated with:

Low-Intensity Exercise for 1 minute consisting of walking on a treadmill at 3 mph.

Repeat for a total of 10 rounds until you reach the 15-minute mark.

Like I mentioned earlier, adjust the intensity of the exercise and the run-walk ratios as needed to accommodate your current fitness level. Maybe you can only run at 7 mph for the first 3 rounds and then you have to go down to 6 mph—that's perfectly fine.

Work on improving on that every time you do the cardio workout. Next time you do the HIIT workout, try to go 4 rounds before you have to go down to 6 mph.

Or maybe you need to walk for longer than a minute in order to fully recuperate; if so, then do it! Remember that, just like with the weight training, the same principle of progressive overload still applies here.

We want to improve our cardiovascular fitness as time goes on.

How to Make HIIT Even More Effective (Yes It's Possible!)

Once you've done the HIIT for 15 minutes, there's something you can do right after that will help to make it even more effective—do 10-15 minutes of slow and steady state cardio immediately after the HIIT.

On its own, slow and steady state cardio isn't the best way to go about things as an endomorph. However, when you combine it with HIIT, something amazing happens.

When you do HIIT, you release free fatty acids into the bloodstream. Then the slow and steady state cardio will come in and burn off those free fatty acids.

If you just do the HIIT, then the free fatty acids will get reabsorbed. That's what makes this combo cardio workout of HIIT and steady state cardio so effective.

To do the steady state cardio, all you need to do is walk at the same pace for 10-15 minutes. For example, on a treadmill, you could walk at a pace of 3 mph for 10-15 minutes and that'll be enough to get the job done.

Here's a breakdown of the entire cardio workout done on a treadmill, which would take you around 25-30 minutes:

Part 1 HIIT:

High-Intensity Exercise for 30 seconds consisting of running on a treadmill at 7 mph.

Alternated with:

Low-Intensity Exercise for 1 minute consisting of walking on a treadmill at 3 mph.

Repeat for a total of 10 rounds until you reach the 15-minute mark.

Part 2 Steady State Cardio:

10-15 minutes of steady state cardio consisting of walking at 3 mph done immediately after the HIIT

Doing this cardio workout 2-3 times per week will be more than enough to start getting you some great results.

What if I Want to Lift Weights and Do Cardio?

Right now you might be wondering what you should do if you want to do both cardio and lift weights. The reality is that you can do cardio by itself or lift weights by itself.

You can do both cardio and lift weights, or you can even not exercise at all. Like I mentioned at the start of this chapter, it's possible to get results solely through your nutrition plan alone.

However, if you do want to lift weights and do cardio, then there's an optimal way to go about it. You have one of two choices—you can do your weight routine and cardio workout on the same day, or you can do them on separate days.

If you choose to do weights and cardio on the same day, then make sure that you do the weight routine first. The reason for this is because if you do cardio first, you may be fatigued, causing you to lift less weight than you normally would have if you were just starting a workout.

Lifting weights first won't cause too much of a performance decrease for your cardio workout. The other option you have is to do these workouts on separate days.

For example, on Mondays, Wednesdays, and Fridays you could lift weights. Then on Tuesdays, Thursdays, and Saturdays you could do cardio.

And if you only wanted to workout five days per week you could do that as well. You could still do the weight routine on Monday, Wednesday, and Friday.

And then you could do the cardio workout on Tuesdays and Thursdays. Do whatever works best for your schedule.

If you find it easy to go to the gym right after work for example, then exercising 5 days per week would be a good way to keep that schedule going. On the other hand, if you have a longer commute to get to the gym, then going less often but doing more when you're there is probably the better way to go.

What About Exercise in a Fasted State?

Fasting is a great and easy nutritional approach to help you burn fat. As it turns out, you can also use fasting to optimize the amount of fat that you burn in the gym.

If you've eaten a meal before working out, your body is in a fed state. This means that the main source of energy your body is going to use to fuel the workout is going to be glycogen.

Of course, if you're a performance athlete this will be beneficial. If you're an average individual who's looking to shed some weight, then we'll want to avoid this if possible.

When you workout in a fasted state, your body will be glycogen depleted. This doesn't mean that your body will totally shut down because it doesn't have any energy to use for the workout.

Instead, your body will have to go somewhere else in order to get the energy it needs to fuel the workout. And that somewhere else is going to be your fat stores.

By working out in a fasted state, you're essentially training your body to become more efficient at using fat for fuel instead of carbs.

Once you finish your workout, what should you do? Most people would say that you need to eat a post workout shake to help your body recover.

If you're an athlete concerned about performance, or someone whose priority is to build muscle, then yes, you should consume a post-workout meal. However, since the main goal is fat loss here, why do you feel obligated to eat something right after you worked out?

I think that the main reason for this is because supplement companies try to shove this idea down our throats. They act as if you have to consume post-workout protein or else your workout was a complete waste, and you're going to lose a lot of muscle.

This couldn't be further from the truth! When you exercise, your growth hormone levels will increase.

The growth hormone will help to save the muscle that you have, plus it'll help you burn more fat. However, when you consume a meal right after your workout, your growth hormone levels will be blunted and your insulin levels will increase.

This will cause you to stop burning fat so your body can instead start to process and store the calories you just ate.

That's why it's actually best if you delay eating anything if possible for 1-2 hours after you finish your workout.

This way you'll be able to take full advantage of the growth hormone increase. Not only that, but think about this logically—how does eating more calories help you lose more weight?

If this is an extra meal you're adding in simply for the sake of eating a post workout shake, how is that going to help you out? It won't!

Now I understand that working out in a fasted state and delaying a meal for 1-2 hours after you finish might not work for your schedule. The ideal way to be able to do this would be to workout early in the morning before you go to work.

If your first meal of the day is at 1:00 p.m. for example, then ideally you'd workout around 10:00 a.m. and finish around 11:00, and then have your meal at 1:00. However, if you can't workout until after you've eaten a meal, then don't sweat it.

Working out in a fasted state is the optimal way to do things for fat loss, but that doesn't mean you're better off not working out at all if you're going to be in a fed state. The same goes for delaying a meal for 1-2 hours after your workout is over.

For example, if you workout at noon and your first meal is usually at one, then go ahead and eat at that time. The main thing I advise against is going out of your way and eating an extra meal at a time when you usually wouldn't eat all because you feel like you have to.

If you finish your workout at a time when you would usually eat anyways, then go ahead and eat at that time.

Can I Add in Calories Burned Through Exercise to My Caloric Calculations?

You might also be wondering about the extra calories you'll be burning through exercise and if you can add those calories to your nutritional calculations. The answer to that is no, you can't.

The reason for this is because I want you to view the calories you burn through exercise as a bonus. These extra calories will either help you reach your goal that much faster or it'll help make up for any potential errors in your calculations.

Most people overestimate the number of calories they burn from exercise as well. This can totally mess up your nutritional calculations.

For example, you might think that you burned off 500 calories in the gym, when in reality you only burned off 250. You'll then eat an extra 250 calories when you shouldn't have, and that can hold you back from making progress.

Therefore, the best thing that you can do is to not factor in calories that you burn from exercise, and instead view them as a bonus.

Chapter 6: What You Need to Do to Ensure the Weight Stays Off

You might have the fear that, even if you are able to lose weight, you'll slowly start to gain it back. In this chapter, I'm going to share with you some tips and strategies you can use to help make sure that once you do lose the weight, it'll stay off for good.

What is Your Goal Bodyweight?

The first thing that you need to figure out is your goal bodyweight. In other words, how much would you ideally want to weigh in order to feel satisfied?

Depending on how far away you are from achieving your goal, you may not know the answer to this. That's completely fine. Most people don't know how much they'd ideally like to weigh.

If this is the case for you, then simply take your best guess as to what you think you'd like to weigh. For example, if someone weighed 230 pounds, he might guess that his goal bodyweight is 170 pounds.

He could then set goals and start to work towards that goal of weighing 170 pounds. As time goes on and he gets closer and closer to his goal, he might realize that his target is off by a bit.

For example, once he gets to 180 pounds he could see that his target bodyweight is better at 175 than 170. Or maybe he gets to 170 and realizes that he be satisfied at 160.

The point is to take your best guess and then adjust as necessary. The only true way to know your goal bodyweight is to look at yourself in the mirror and see if you're happy with how you look.

If you are, then step on the scale and see how much you weigh. That's your goal bodyweight.

Obviously, you don't have a crystal ball to see what that number is, so take your best guess with where you're at right now. You can always adjust it later as you start making progress.

What Should You Do When You Reach Your Target Bodyweight?

When you do reach your goal bodyweight, how do things change? Should you keep doing things exactly as you were to lose weight in the first place?

Or should you go back to your old eating habits? As you can probably guess, you shouldn't go back to your old eating patterns.

Doing so will cause you to gain back the weight that you worked so hard to lose in the first place. Instead, you should continue eating in the same way that you did to lose the weight in the first place.

However, you won't be eating the same amount of calories. Let's say for example you were eating 2,200 calories per day in order to lose 1 pound per week.

Now that you've reached your goal bodyweight, you no longer need to continue eating in a caloric deficit. You're now going to eat at your maintenance caloric intake.

This is because you now want to maintain your new bodyweight instead of continuing to lose weight. To figure out what your current maintenance calories are, simply find out how large of a deficit your were creating and add that number back to your current caloric intake.

For example, if you were eating 2,200 calories a day in order to lose 1 pound per week, this would mean that you were eating at a deficit of 500 calories per day. You would simply take 2,200 and add 500 to that number to reach 2,700 calories per day.

This is how many calories you'll need to eat every day to maintain your new bodyweight. This is pretty cool!

You now get to enjoy eating some more calories without having to worry about the weight coming back. You still want to be mindful of how much you're eating though.

It can be easy to get carried away and overeat. That's why you want to make sure that you're still measuring your calories and macros.

With that being said, what's the best way to go about adding in those additional calories? It's not wise to add an additional meal to your diet plan.

For example, if you're currently eating 3 meals per day, then stick with that. Don't bump that up to 4 meals per day.

The reason for this is because those extra calories might not be enough to justify eating another meal. This might cause you to overeat, and we want to avoid that at all costs.

Instead, a better idea is to add more to the meals that you're currently eating. For example, you could eat an additional side dish for one of your meals.

Or you could eat 250 calories more of a side dish for two of your meals. You can break it up however you like as long as you're accurately accounting for everything that you eat.

And like I mentioned earlier, your eating patterns need to stay the same. This means that if you were fasting for 16 hours a day, eating a moderate amount of carbs, and eating healthy foods 85% of the time, then you need to continue doing those things.

If you start to deviate from what made you successful in the first place, then you'll start gaining the weight back. This is why sustainability is key.

If it's too hard to follow a diet plan, you won't be able to maintain your goal bodyweight. This endomorph nutrition plan is set up in a way to make it easy for you to continue the plan once you're satisfied with where you're at.

At the end of the day, you need to remember that you must make some sort of sacrifice in order to get results and keep them. You can't be sedentary, eat what you want, when you want to, in any amount that you want and expect to be happy with your fitness results.

A sacrifice has to be made somewhere. The more willing you are to make sacrifices, the better off you'll be. You don't need to go crazy, but there has to be some give somewhere.

With this diet plan, we're sacrificing when you can eat, and the overall amount that you can eat for the day. This is the easiest thing to surrender.

You don't have to completely give up certain foods, and you don't have to exercise if you don't want to. Do take note that, even though this nutrition plan is made to be as easy as possible, it still requires you to give up some things in order to get you to where you want to go.

Make no mistake about it, getting in shape requires discipline and effort for a prolonged period of time.

Chapter 7: Endomorph Supplement Guide

In this chapter, I'm going to share with you everything you need to know about supplements. Supplements are a very popular topic among fitness enthusiasts, but it's also a confusing one.

By the end of this chapter, you'll know exactly what supplements can help you out along the way and which ones you should avoid. Let's get started...

The Correct Way to Think About Supplements

The supplement industry is a multibillion-dollar industry. That sure is a lot of money, and sadly, a lot of supplement companies may not have your best interest at heart.

They might try to sell you on something that isn't backed by very much research and is mostly hype. And if you aren't properly educated on supplements, it can be very easy to fall for the hype.

This is why it's so critical that you think of supplements in the correct way. What is a supplement anyway?

It's meant to be a tool that enhances something when the supplement is added to it. For example, a supplement is meant to enhance a proper exercise and nutrition plan.

However, most people don't view supplements in this manner. Instead, they view supplements as something that is meant to replace a proper diet and exercise routine.

As if the supplement can do all of the work for them. And this isn't uncommon.

Most people who buy weight loss supplements aren't doing it to supplement a proper nutrition plan. Instead, they're hoping to lose weight without having to put forth any effort, similar to a get rich quick scheme.

Like I said, billions of dollars are being made here and yet the obesity epidemic is only getting worse. It can be so easy to fall for the magical hype of a new weight loss supplement.

You'll see a commercial for a new weight loss pill, and you'll see all of these people who supposedly lost weight using it. So you buy into it, all while ignoring the little asterisk on the bottom of the screen that says something like "participants used this pill alongside a proper diet and exercise plan."

That's why the first lesson you need to understand when it comes to supplements is that there is nothing magical about them. They're meant to add to a proper diet and exercise plan, not replace them.

At the end of the day, it's still going to require dedicated effort and persistence in order to reach your goals. There is no getting around that. Supplement companies know that you have to work hard to reach your goals, but they prey on people who want to take a shortcut.

People will wonder what the harm is in trying the product; it's only $20. If it doesn't work, then I lose $20, but if it does work, then I'll get in shape without having to put forth any effort.

The reward greatly outweighs the risk. This is a similar mentality people have when playing the lottery.

Even though the odds of you winning are extremely slim, millions of people still play the lottery every year for the hope that they can get rich without having to work for it. The risk of wasting $2 on a lottery ticket is well worth the potential reward of winning millions, even if that chance is quite slim.

The second thing you need to understand about supplements is that no supplement is required in order for you to reach your fitness goal. If someone says that supplement x is a must-have in order to lose weight, then they're not telling the truth.

The truth is that you don't need any supplements in order to get in better shape. I want you to be able to experience this truth first hand.

That's why for the first 6 weeks that you're doing the diet program, you're not allowed to take any supplements. I want you to see that it is possible to get results without having to take any supplements.

Then once that 6-week period is up, you can take some of the supplements that I'll recommend later in the chapter. This is a great way to go about doing things because you'll get into the habit of following the nutrition plan before taking any supplements.

Most people do the exact opposite of this. They decide that they want to start a new fitness routine.

Then they immediately go to the supplement store and buy a bunch of supplements before they've actually even started their plan! Then time goes by and they never get around to starting their nutrition plan and the supplements sit there and collect dust.

Doing things the other way around proves to yourself that you're dedicated enough to actually get some benefits out of supplements if you use them. This should come as a relief.

You don't have to worry about spending extra money on supplements if you don't want to, or if you don't have room in your budget for them. Usually, it's the simplest things that work best, such as eating right and exercising.

However, that doesn't necessarily mean simple is easy. The third tip when it comes to supplements is to buy what you can afford in terms of importance.

While you may not want to completely skip out on supplements, you might only be able to afford one supplement. That's completely fine.

Don't feel as if you have to buy multiple supplements in order for them to be worth it. I'll be sharing with you the benefits of different popular supplements and which ones to get first if you're on a limited budget.

Finally, if everything else is in order, what kind of a difference can you expect supplements to make? I'd say that the right supplements, when paired in conjunction with a good diet plan, could make around a 5-10% difference at most.

So you can look at that however you like. You certainly can't get around the fact that 90-95% of your results are coming from your nutrition and exercise plan.

However, if you want that last little boost, supplements could be the thing to help you get there. With that being said, let's get into what supplements are worth your money and which ones aren't...

Supplements You Should Avoid

Here are some popular supplements that you should avoid at all costs, even though they're quite popular. Don't buy into the hype with these supplements because they're just that—hype!

Testosterone boosters

Testosterone is a male sex hormone that is responsible for sex drive, strength, muscle size, bone mass, and distribution of fat. This isn't to say that only men have testosterone; women have testosterone too.

However, women have much less testosterone than men do. With all of these benefits, it's easy to see why testosterone boosters are a very popular supplement for men.

The way this supplement is presented makes people think that they can get similar benefits to steroids without any negative consequences. The truth is that this supplement is a bunch of hype and not much more.

Most testosterone boosters will use one or more of the following ingredients—ZMA, D-aspartic acid, and tribulus terrestris. The research shows that at best D-aspartic acid can temporarily increase testosterone levels (4).

Multiple studies show that tribulus terrestris doesn't have any effect on testosterone levels (5). What tribulus terrestris will do is increase libido, which will make you think that the supplement is really working.

ZMA is only effective at increasing testosterone levels if you're deficient in zinc to begin with (6). Testosterone boosters aren't a good route to go if you want to increase your testosterone levels.

However, there are a few things you can do if you want to naturally increase your testosterone levels. The first is to improve your body composition.

There's a correlation between body composition levels and testosterone. Correlation doesn't mean causation. However, as you start to lean down, this should mean your testosterone levels will start to go up some.

The other thing that you can do is regularly lift weights, as this has been shown to help increase testosterone levels as well (7). You're going to be following a sound nutrition plan and exercise plan if you choose to exercise.

Therefore, you really have nothing to worry about in regards to your testosterone levels. Just focus on the main task at hand, which is reaching your goal bodyweight, and you'll be good to go.

Fat Burners

Most fat burner supplements are a waste of your money. It's a little ironic that a supplement specifically designed to help you lose weight fails miserably at what it's supposed to do.

They'll use a variety of different ingredients that are allegedly going to help you boost your metabolism and suppress your appetite, among other claims. Here are some of the ingredients you may find in fat burners, and why they're not effective at what they claim to do:

Hoodia

This comes from a desert cactus in countries in Africa. It's supposed to help blunt your appetite, therefore allowing you to lose weight because you wouldn't be eating as much.

However, hoodia is not only ineffective at suppressing your appetite, it can also be harmful to your body by causing an increase in blood pressure (8).

Vitamin B12

This is a vitamin that helps to convert foods we eat into energy and it helps with the formation of red blood cells. Some claim that B12 can help to increase weight loss because of the boost in energy that it can provide.

However, this may only be the case for individuals who have a deficiency in vitamin B12 to begin with. There's not sufficient evidence to show that taking more B12 is beneficial to weight loss for individuals who already have normal B12 levels (9).

Garcinia Cambogia

This ingredient comes from the tropical fruit tamarind. It's supposed to help limit the production of fat in the body and suppress appetite.

However, there's not conclusive evidence to help support that these claims are anything more than temporary at best (10).

BCAA's

If you're going to be working out in a fasted state, then you may feel the need to buy BCAA's. The main selling point behind them is that they can help prevent excessive muscle breakdown during your workouts.

I almost fell for the hype on this supplement back in college, but fortunately they were too expensive, and I couldn't afford to waste my money on them! BCAA's stand for branch chained amino acids, and they're essentially the broken down form of protein.

This allows them to be more easily digested and utilized by the body faster than protein. Eating food before you train spikes your insulin; however, amino acids have a much smaller impact on your insulin levels.

Therefore, you can take amino acids before your workout and still train in a fasted state. The amino acid leucine is the most effective one at preventing muscle breakdown.

However, you have to think about the cost here. Is it really worth investing in amino acids (which can be quite expensive) to ensure you're not losing muscle?

Remember, if you're already eating an adequate amount of protein every day and you're not super lean to begin with, then your body will want to use fat for fuel instead of protein (i.e. your muscle).

If you're already very lean and not getting in a lot of protein, then BCAA's probably would be worth it if you're exercising in a fasted state. For most people though, it's not going to be worth the money.

Pre Workout Supplements

This is another supplement that's extremely popular nowadays. The idea behind this supplement is that it'll help to increase the intensity of your workouts, allowing you to burn more calories and lose more weight.

Yes, most pre-workout supplements do contain some beneficial ingredients such as citrulline malate, but again is it worth the cost, especially considering what your goals are? The reason why I say this is because you could be paying for ingredients that help you increase muscle size and strength, like creatine.

Creatine is a great supplement, but if your main goal is fat loss, do you really want to pay for something that won't help you reach your primary goal? Additionally, pre-workout supplements commonly contain arginine AKG (AAKG) which helps to provide better blood flow to the muscles.

In the fitness world, this is referred to as getting a pump. You don't have to get a pump to gain strength or build muscle, and you certainly don't need to get a pump to burn fat.

It may look and feel good, but its tangible benefits are questionable. Not only that, but do you want to become reliant on something in order to have a good workout?

Imagine that you're about to go to the gym, but then you realize you're out of your pre-workout supplement, so you decide to workout later after you can go to the store. Chances are good that you'll never get around to completing that workout.

You're now relying on your pre-workout supplement as a crutch, and it'll start dictating how good your workouts are, or if they will even happen in the first place. Even with this being the case, you still might be interested in taking something like a pre-workout.

There's a much cheaper option that I'll be sharing with you in the recommended supplements section. This will provide you with many of the same benefits that the expensive pre-workout supplements will at only a fraction of the cost.

Multivitamins

Maybe you're like me and you grew up taking a multivitamin with breakfast. My chewable multivitamin tasted good, and my mom told me it would help me stay healthy so I actually enjoyed taking it.

Now though, there are much better things I'd rather spend my money on. A multivitamin contains of a bunch of different micronutrients.

These are things our bodies need in small amounts in order to survive. Conversely, macronutrients like protein, carbs, and fat are things our bodies need in large amounts in order to properly function.

This is what makes multivitamins seem like they're such a great supplement. All you have to do is take a pill and it'll help make up for any vitamin deficiencies that you may have.

This begs the question of whether or not most people are deficient with a lot of the vitamins contained in these multivitamin pills? Are we once again being sold something that we don't really need?

Some multivitamins will claim that they can help prevent certain diseases or illnesses like cardiovascular disease. However, you have to consider how healthy the individual is to begin with.

Someone who's already eating a healthy diet and exercising regularly isn't going to need a multivitamin to help prevent certain diseases. On the other hand, someone who's nutrient deficient would need to take in more of certain vitamins and minerals.

Then again, is a multivitamin the best way to go about doing this? It would be better if the person instead focused on improving his or her diet by eating more wholesome foods.

Not only would this save you money, but consuming vitamins and minerals from whole food sources is better absorbed by the body than consuming them via a pill. Most individuals in counties where there is an overabundance of food are probably not deficient in most of the vitamins that are contained in a multivitamin pill.

Therefore, multivitamins aren't worth it for most people. The body will simply secrete most of the excess not needed through urine.

Not only that but taking a multivitamin might make you feel as if it's okay for you to eat more junk food than you should because the multivitamin will help make up for it. If you follow the nutrition principles as they're laid out in this book, then you shouldn't have any need for a multivitamin.

Sadly, the multivitamin supplement is something a lot of people fall for because it makes us feel better about ourselves. It makes us feel like we're taking a proactive step in taking care of our health.

And depending on how deficient you are, then maybe you actually could be. Chances are good though that the multivitamin pill isn't benefiting you much, and your money would be better spent elsewhere.

Digestive Enzymes

This is a supplement that I've recommended in the past, however upon further study I've realized that this supplement is meant more for specific individuals with digestive problems, such as irritable bowel syndrome.

Taking digestive enzymes won't be worth it for most people. Enzymes are found in certain foods (such as fruits and vegetables) and they're produced by the body.

Whenever we eat food, enzymes will help to break down the food so that the body can absorb it. For example, protein will get broken down into amino acids, carbs will get broken down into glucose, and fat will get broken down into fatty acids.

Our bodies have specific enzymes that help to break down each of these macronutrients and many others. The idea behind taking the supplement is that it can help you absorb more of the nutrients from the foods that you're eating.

This is important because what you eat technically isn't as important as what you absorb. Remember that your body releases the enzymes necessary to break down the foods that you're eating.

If you're getting your enzymes from an outside supplement, then over time your body will stop naturally producing enzymes because it no longer needs to. This is similar to when a male takes steroids to boost testosterone.

Over time the testes will stop naturally producing testosterone because the body is getting sufficient amounts from an outside source. If you're not currently suffering from any digestive issues, then the best thing you can do to maximize enzyme production and help improve your digestive health is to slow down and chew your food properly.

Most people only chew their food 3-4 times before swallowing. This is a problem because as you chew, your body releases enzymes to help your body digest that food.

If you don't spend enough time properly chewing your food, then you're not giving your body much of a chance to release the necessary enzymes to break down that food. Instead, you want to chew slowly and enough times to where the food is almost liquidly before you swallow.

This means you'll chew your food around 30 times before swallowing. Not only will this help improve your digestion, but it can also help you lose more weight by consuming less food.

When you eat faster, you might wind up consuming more calories because it can take 20 minutes from the time you start eating for the stomach to signal to the brain that you're full and to stop eating. Therefore, most people are better off slowing down and properly chewing their food rather than taking a digestive enzyme.

Detox Supplements

This is a supplement that's been gaining a lot of popularity in recent years. The selling point is that your body contains a lot of toxins that need to be dispelled of.

By using a special detox kit, you can help to cleanse your body of harmful toxins that are holding you back from losing weight. The problem is that different detox supplements are made by different companies, and these companies can't seem to agree on exactly what a toxin is.

This makes it hard to know what the supplement is trying to get rid of and how it's getting rid of it. Some detox supplements contain a polymerizing agent that causes your poop to stick together.

This can cause you to excrete one large piece of stool when you use the bathroom. This may lead you to think the supplement is really making a difference, when it reality it isn't doing anything to truly help you.

This might be the reason why some people claim that they feel better after going on a detox. The truth is that it could very well be a placebo instead of something the supplement actually did.

Your body is already set up with organs like the liver and kidneys that are designed to help filter and get rid of waste in the body. This isn't to say you should go wild and overload these organs by eating junk food all of the time, or excessively drink and smoke.

Instead, you can help support these organs in your body by living a proper healthy lifestyle. You can do this by making sure that you're eating lots of wholesome foods, getting plenty of sleep, and exercising.

Supplements That Are Worth Your Money

Now it's time to get into what you should be buying if you want to invest some money into supplements. They're going to be listed in order of importance; however, certain supplements may suit your individual needs better.

At the end of the day, I recommend going with what will best fit your budget and your needs.

Protein Powder

The first supplement that I would recommend getting is protein powder. The reason for it is rather simple—convenience.

Having protein powder makes it so much easier to reach your daily protein intake. Not only that, but if you find yourself in a pinch without any healthy foods to eat, protein powder can be an easy way to consume quality calories.

Make no mistake about it, there's nothing special about the protein that's in protein powder. It's simply protein in a powder form.

This is true regardless of what various supplement companies will tell you. The main thing you want to focus on is making sure you're getting an adequate amount of protein.

Sometimes it can be hard to reach your daily protein macros solely from whole food sources. Ideally, you'd get all the protein you need from whole foods.

When you can't though, this is where protein powder really shines. You can easily make a protein shake or mix the powder in with some other food like cottage cheese or plain greek yogurt.

This can be part of a healthy high protein meal. Compare this to eating protein from whole foods, such as lean meats like chicken or beef.

You have to buy the meat, then prepare it, cook it, eat it, and clean up afterwards. If you find yourself in a pinch for time, or maybe you're away from your house, then protein powder will come in handy.

The thing you want to watch out for is something known as protein guilt. This is where you consume more protein than necessary for fear of losing muscle, or because you think that you have to eat a certain amount of protein with every meal.

Remember that the goal is to lose weight. Consuming more calories than necessary (even if they're from protein) will take you farther away from your goal, not closer to it.

Of course, 40% of your total calories will be coming from protein, so it's unlikely that you'll overeat it. Regardless, it's still something you want to be aware of.

Not all protein powder is created equally though. You'll definitely want to make sure that you get the correct protein powder to help suit your needs.

The first thing you need to find out is what type of protein powder you'll want to get. Whey protein is the most common type of protein on the market.

It's a milk-based type of protein and it tends to be the cheapest type of protein you can buy. There are many other different kinds of protein powder such as soy, beef, hemp, egg, and pea protein, among others.

Unless you have some type of allergy to dairy or you're lactose intolerant, then sticking with whey protein is going to be your best bet. If you do have an allergy or are lactose intolerant, then going with something like an egg protein would probably be your best option.

Yes, this is going to be more expensive than something like a whey protein, but it's a very high-quality type of protein that you'll be able to consume without issues. As far as whey protein is concerned, there are three main kinds that you can get—concentrate, isolate, and hydrolysate.

Whey concentrate is the cheapest of the three kinds. This is because whey concentrate contains a lower percentage of protein than the other two kinds.

A good concentrate will contain around 70-80% of the total calories per serving from protein. The rest will be made up of carbs and fat. This is the type of protein that I've used for years, and it's worked great for me.

The other two types of whey protein may suit your needs better though. The next type of whey protein is whey isolate.

Whey isolate contains a higher percentage of protein and fewer carbs and fat. Typically, whey isolate contains around 90% of the total calories per serving from protein, which is pretty good.

If you're willing to pay a bit more money, this could be a better option for you, especially if you want to avoid the extra carbs and fat the concentrate contains.

Finally, we have whey hydrolysate. This is the most expensive of the three kinds of whey protein. It's a predigested protein which means that it'll get absorbed by the body the fastest.

This may be something to consider if your primary goal is to build muscle; however, it won't serve much of a use for fat loss purposes, especially for how much more expensive it is.

When you're looking to buy a protein powder, there are some things that you're going to want to watch out for. This will mostly apply for when you're looking to buy a whey concentrate protein powder.

Be that as it may, it still doesn't hurt to double check these things when buying an isolate or hydrolysate protein. The first thing you want to check is the ingredient list.

The first ingredient on the label should be protein or protein blend. That may seem obvious, but that isn't always the case with some protein powders.

Some protein powders are made with cheap fillers such as maltodextrin. If something like maltodextrin is the first ingredient on the label, then you should avoid buying that protein powder.

The next thing you want to be on the lookout for is something known as a proprietary blend. You may notice the words proprietary blend on the nutrition info on the protein powder.

The specific amount of any ingredient listed under the proprietary blend doesn't have to be listed. For someone who knows what to look for, this definitely makes it seem like the company is trying to hide something.

The proprietary blend could list mostly high-quality ingredients and one cheap filler ingredient. Since the amount isn't listed, the blend could consist mostly of that one cheap ingredient and you'd have no way of knowing.

And since most people don't know what a proprietary blend is, this will even get marketed as a good thing sometimes. Some companies will try to use the proprietary blend to help increase the perceived value of their product.

When you see the words 'proprietary blend' on a protein powder label, you should not buy that protein. There's simply no way to tell if something is trying to be covered up.

A reputable company won't try to hide any of their ingredients or the amounts of those ingredients that are contained in their protein powder. The next thing you'll want to check for is the percentage of protein the powder contains.

If you're buying a whey protein concentrate, then you want to make sure the protein contains no less than 70% of the total calories per serving from protein. Ideally, this number would be 80%, but as long as it's 70% and above, you'll be okay.

Anything lower than 70% means that you're not getting your money's worth. You're likely paying for cheap filler carbs that aren't going to help you reach your goal.

To figure this out, look at the nutritional info and see how many calories per serving the powder contains. Then look at the serving size for the protein, which is typically going to be in grams.

Take that number and multiply it by four to convert it into calories. Then divide the protein calories by the total calories to get your percentage. For example:

220 total calories per serving

40 grams of protein per serving

40x4=160

160/220= .73 which converts to 73%

This means that this protein powder contains 73% of the total calories from protein, so it passes the test. The last thing that you want to look out for is something known as amino acid spiking.

This is where companies will spike their formulas with cheap amino acids in order to get a higher protein reading during testing. This allows them to get away with putting higher amounts of protein on the label than the powder actually contains.

Of course, companies aren't going to blatantly put on their label that they spike their formula. Therefore, it's up to you to do your own research and make sure that you're buying from a trustworthy company.

Ultimately, if a protein powder passes all of these four tests, then it's a good protein powder and worth buying. Yes, there is quite a bit to look out for when it comes to buying protein, but doing your homework will pay off.

Protein powder is one of the most popular supplements out there. That kind of status attracts companies who will do shady things in order to get your money.

Fish Oil

The next supplement on the recommended list is going to be fish oil. There are two different kinds of essential fatty acids—Omega 6 and Omega 3 fatty acids.

Our bodies don't make these fatty acids, so we must consume them through our diets. Omega 6 fatty acids are an inflammatory fatty acid.

This aspect of Omega 6's isn't bad in and of itself. In fact, it's important for a properly functioning immune system.

The problem occurs when things get out of balance and we consume too many Omega 6's in comparison to Omega 3's. Foods that are commonly high in Omega 6 fatty acids include various types of nuts such as walnuts and different oils like soybean oil.

Omega 3 fatty acids, on the other hand, act as an anti-inflammatory in the body. These are found commonly in foods such as fish, chia seeds, and flax seeds.

Anti-inflammatories are important for preventing chronic diseases. In fact, any disease that ends in the suffix -itis is caused by an excessive amount of inflammation in a certain area. For example, arthritis is an inflammation of the joints.

Omega 3 fatty acids can help improve heart health; research has shown that Omega 3 fatty acids can increase HDL cholesterol, which is the good kind of cholesterol.

Some studies also show that supplementing with Omega 3's can help boost your metabolism (11). However, this is a slight boost at best, and it's definitely nothing that will be able to replace a proper diet and exercise routine.

The main reason to supplement with fish oil isn't for any potential weight loss benefits. It's more so for your overall health.

Most Americans consume way more Omega 6 fatty acids than Omega 3 fatty acids; this is where problems can arise. By supplementing with Omega 3 fatty acids, you'll help close that gap and keep your body from becoming chronically inflamed.

This will allow you to stay healthy and be able to focus your attention on your weight loss goals. It's hard to do that if you're feeling sick.

As with most supplements, quality is going to be key here. A lot of the fish oils on the market are low grade and aren't going to be worth your money.

So what should you look out for when buying this supplement? The first thing is going to be how the oil is being extracted from the fish during the manufacturing process.

You want to make sure the supplement uses cold pressed manufacturing techniques in order to extract the oil. Cheaper fish oils that use heat to extract the oil from the fish can lead to oxidative damage.

This can cause more inflammation to arise in your body, which defeats the purpose of taking the supplement in the first place. The next thing you want to make sure of is that the fish used were caught from the wild and not from farm-raised fish.

Wild fish will be of a better quality than farm-raised fish. Thirdly, you want to check to make sure that the fish oil supplement is certified for purity by a third party.

You don't want the fish oil to contain an excessive amount of toxins. Ideally, a fish oil supplement should contain no more than 100 parts per billion mercury, 100 parts per billion PCB's, 100 parts per billion arsenic, and 2 parts per trillion dioxins and furans.

Finally, you want to check how much EPA and DHA are contained in the supplement. EPA and DHA are the main Omega 3 fatty acids that you're after.

Some fish oil supplements will be sneaky and say that their supplement contains 1,000 mg of fish oil per serving. Yet the total EPA and DHA might only be 250 mg of that 1,000 mg.

Essentially, the total amount of fish oil per serving doesn't matter. You should instead focus on how much EPA and DHA the supplement contains. That's why you must carefully read the label before buying.

Ideally, you want to aim for around 1,800 to 3,000 mg of EPA and DHA per day depending on your needs. This is a total amount between the two, not a recommendation for each one.

For example, if you were taking 1,800 mg daily, you might consume 900 mg of EPA's and 900 mg of DHA's. Of course, this doesn't all have to come from supplementation.

You can get some or all of your Omega 3's from your diet. It's similar to the protein powder.

If you find it hard to get an adequate amount of Omega 3's in your diet, then consider supplementing with them for the sake of convenience.

You may also be wondering about krill oil; it is quite similar to fish oil in the sense that it's an Omega 3 supplement that contains EPA's and DHA's. However, there are a few differences between the two.

For starters, krill oil contains the antioxidant known as astaxanthin, which is rarely found in fish oil. Antioxidants are important for combating free radicals, improving skin health, and supporting a healthy immune system, among other things.

These are some great benefits; however, that's about the only major benefit you'll get from taking krill oil over fish oil. Thanks to the marketing around astaxanthin, krill oil tends to be more expensive per serving than fish oil does.

Not only that, but many krill oils actually contain less EPA's and DHA's per serving than fish oils do! This isn't always the case, but always make sure you check the labels before you buy.

If you have to spend more money to get an adequate amount of EPA's and DHA's, then it's not worth it. You're taking the supplement for the EPA's and the DHA's, not to get the antioxidant astaxanthin.

If you want to get more antioxidants in your body, then eat more foods such as blueberries, strawberries, walnuts, and kale.

Caffeine

The last recommended supplement on the list is also the cheapest—caffeine. Caffeine can help to give you a boost in energy by blocking a neurotransmitter known as adenosine.

This boost in energy can help increase exercise intensity, allowing you to burn more calories at the gym. This is the better pre-workout supplement that I alluded to earlier and the reason why is simple.

Caffeine gives you very similar benefits to that of a pre-workout, yet it's only a fraction of the cost per serving. You can drink coffee or even take it in the form of a caffeine pill before your workout to help increase performance.

There is also some research out there to show that caffeine can help to boost your metabolism (12). However, don't expect anything too crazy from this.

Remember that supplements only make a small difference when paired in conjunction with a proper diet and exercise plan. Everyone would be in great shape if all you had to do was drink coffee before heading off to work.

Finally, if you're already a coffee drinker, I want to advise that you to stick as closely to pure black coffee as you can. The more sugar, creamer, and milk you add to the coffee, the worse off the beverage is going to be for you.

Any boost in metabolism the coffee does provide to you will quickly be erased by the extra calories you're consuming, thus defeating the purpose.

You probably noticed that the list of recommended supplements was much shorter than the list you should avoid. That wasn't by accident; most supplements on the market aren't that good.

And the ones that I do recommend aren't going to be able to do all of the work for you. Don't ever get mistaken by the fact that most of the time supplements sell because of hype and the hope that they might work.

It can be easy to fall for the latest craze of a new supplement that just hit the market. However, the vast majority of new supplements that come out aren't going to be worth it.

So if you're interested in checking out a new supplement, use the test of time. See how the long the supplement has been around for.

For example, protein powder has been around for a while, and it's not going anywhere anytime soon. On the other hand, if a brand new fat burner came out last week, hold off on buying it.

See if it'll still be around 3-5 years later and if there is science is to back it up. The test of time doesn't guarantee a supplement to be worth it, but it's a good place to start.

At the end of the day, make sure that you always do a thorough amount of research on the supplement and the brand before you buy.

Chapter 8: Frequently Asked Questions

What Can I Drink While I'm Fasting?

When you're fasting, you should only drink beverages that contain zero calories. Most of the time, this means that you're going to be drinking water, which is how it should be.

You can always use a water enhancer to add a little flavor to the water if you prefer that. Aside from water, black coffee and green tea are also an option for you to drink during your fasting periods.

The main thing is that the drink does not contain any calories. If it does, that drink can break your fast, and we don't want that to happen.

Drinking diet sodas would therefore be acceptable, however, I recommend avoiding them if possible. Diet soda contains artificial sweeteners like aspartame and saccharin in them.

There's also research to show that diet soda may spark dopamine in the brain and fuel hormones that cause hunger (13). This can lead to an increase in appetite.

That's something you'll definitely want to avoid when you're trying to fast for a certain length of time. You may drink diet soda and not notice any difference in your appetite. Even if this is the case, it is clear that diet soda does not provide your diet any nutritional value.

That's why you should stick with water as much as possible, even if the taste is bland. If you're currently drinking a lot of soda right now, do your best to slowly wean yourself off of it.

Don't try to quit cold turkey. If you try to do that, it'll make things feel overwhelming, and most likely cause you to start drinking them again.

For example, if you're drinking 20 ounces of soda per day, start by trying to scale that back to 16 ounces per day. Then a week later, go down to 12 ounces; continue this pattern until you get to zero.

Drinking 20 ounces of soda per day is around 240 calories and 65 grams of sugar! And since those are empty calories, they aren't going to do anything to help keep you full.

They're simply going to take away from other foods that you could be eating. That's why it's really important to get to the point where you're drinking water the majority of the time.

How Many Meals Should I Eat Per Day?

There's a myth that eating 6 small meals throughout the day will help to boost your metabolism. Research shows that meal frequency does not affect weight loss (14).

This means that it doesn't matter whether you eat 6 meals, 3 meals, or just one meal a day; your weight loss will not be affected as long as you're still eating the same overall amount of calories.

This means that you can eat however many meals a day that works best for you and your schedule. Since you're going to be doing the fasting protocol, this means you're probably going to be eating 2 or 3 meals per day.

Doing anything more than that will be hard to squeeze into an eight-hour feeding window. In addition to that, the meals would likely be so small that they might not fill you up very well.

Eating fewer meals will allow you to eat larger and more satisfying meals. It's up to you if you'd rather eat two or three meals a day.

In an earlier chapter, I gave the example of fasting until noon and then eating three meals—one at noon, one at 4:00, and one at 8:00. If you prefer, you could eat only two meals during that eight-hour feeding window instead of three.

For example, you could eat at noon and 6:00 p.m, or maybe 1:00 p.m. and 7:00 p.m.

You can break it up however you like. When you eat, you might enjoy feasting on larger meals, in which case 2 meals per day would be more up your alley.

Or maybe you're able to better control how much you eat if you consume 3 meals a day. Again, simply do whatever works best for you and your schedule.

How Should You Divide Up Calories Across Your Meals?

Let's say you're eating 2,100 calories per day across 3 meals in order to lose weight. You might think that you need to eat 700 calories per meal, but you certainly don't have to do things that way if you don't want to.

You can divide up your calories across your meals in whatever way that you like. For example, if you usually don't like eating that big of a lunch, you could eat a smaller lunch and save some of those extra calories for later in the day during dinner.

Your first meal could contain 400 calories, your second meal 1,000, and your final meal 700. This still works out to the same 2,100 calorie total for the day.

The point is to break things up in a way that works best for you and your schedule. Remember, we're focused on the long haul here.

If it's easier for you to eat more calories during one meal and less during another, then definitely do that!

What Should I Do If I Find It Hard to Adapt to Fasting When I First Start?

When most people first start fasting, they find it to be rather difficult. This should come as no surprise because most of us have been eating breakfast our whole lives.

Our bodies have been trained to expect a meal in the morning soon after we wake up. However, if our bodies can be trained to expect a meal soon after waking, then that means we can also train our bodies to expect the first meal to come later in the day.

While this initial transition period may not be fun, think of what will happen when you make it to the other side. You'll be used to delaying your first meal of the day, and you'll be able to fast with ease.

In fact, it really won't feel like a diet at that point. It would be harder to quit and go back to eating breakfast than it would be to continue skipping it.

With that being said though, how do you reach that point? Well, the first thing you need to understand is that it can take about 2-4 weeks in order for you to fully adapt to your new fasting protocol.

This is definitely something you'll want to keep in mind. Initially, when you're first starting out, you might want to quit because it seems like this will never end.

However, it will end. The hunger you're feeling will only be temporary.

Once you make it to the other side, those feelings of hunger in the morning will stop persisting. Therefore, always keep in mind that you can do this for 2-4 weeks, and you'll be good to go for a very long time to come. It won't last forever.

Aside from that mental tip, the first thing you want to make sure you're doing is drinking enough water upon waking up. The reason for this is because you haven't had any water during the night while you were sleeping.

This means that you're going to be dehydrated when you wake up. Sometimes our bodies will confuse our dehydration with hunger.

This is known as false hunger. There's a chance that you could be eating breakfast when you're not even actually hungry—you could simply be dehydrated!

That's why it's critical that you drink a couple of glasses of water as soon as you can after waking up. Even after that, make sure you're drinking plenty of water throughout the day.

The best way to be able to tell if you're dehydrated or not is to go by the color of your urine. If your urine is more of a yellow color, then that means you're dehydrated.

If it's clear, you're hydrated. This is the first step you need to take in order to make adapting to fasting easier.

Sadly, even though everyone wakes up dehydrated, most people still don't drink nearly enough water in the morning or throughout the day! After that, the next thing you may want to consider doing is drinking black coffee.

Coffee can help to blunt your appetite, and it can also help to give you a small boost in metabolism as I mentioned earlier. Even if you're not a regular coffee drinker, this may be something you'll want to try if you notice that it makes the adjustment phase easier.

Finally, the last thing you can do if you notice that you're hungry before it's time to eat is to chew gum. Make sure that the gum is sugar-free, and that it contains 5 or fewer calories.

We don't want to consume anything that could break our fast earlier than wanted, which includes chewing gum. You might not think that chewing gum would do much, but it surprisingly does.

The first reason why it helps so much is because it distracts you. You're not focusing as much on your hunger as you are on chewing the gum.

Not only that, but you can't eat anything if you have a piece of gum in your mouth. Yes, you could simply spit the gum out and eat something, but for some weird reason you might find that you won't want to eat anything until you're done chewing the piece of gum.

Psychologically, this could be because of something that is known as a sunk cost. You spent money on the gum, and you want to get the maximum value out of it.

You don't want to feel as if you wasted your money on gum that you barely chewed. If you spat it out after 5 minutes to eat something, then it wouldn't feel like you got much value out of it.

That's why chewing gum can be so powerful. You just have to get started with it, and it could be 30 minutes before you're ready to spit it out.

And by that point, you may have forgotten that you're even hungry! Finally, once you're done chewing the gum, you're going to have a minty fresh breath that you may not be so eager to ruin by eating something.

Yes, chewing gum may be a sneaky little tactic, but do whatever tricks work in the beginning to get the job done.

The last thing you want to make sure you're doing is keeping yourself busy. Distract yourself however you can.

The more bored you are, the more your mind is going to remind you of how hungry you are. Think of a time in the past, a time when you did something so fun that you forgot to eat for hours.

That's what I'm talking about here. The more you can keep your mind engaged at work or with your family, the better off you'll be.

Initially, when you first start fasting, this might mean planning some fun activities to do with your friends or family on the weekend. You don't want to sit around bored with nothing to do on the weekends.

This might cause you to eat simply because you were bored, and you didn't have anything better to do. Remember, you just have to survive for 2-4 weeks until you make it to the other side. It'll be well worth it when you do!

How Much Water Should I Drink Per Day?

The next thing you might be wondering is how much water you should be drinking per day in order to stay hydrated. The standard answer is that you should drink eight, eight-ounce glasses of water throughout the day.

However, this is a blanket answer that doesn't suit individual needs. For example, this would have a 5-foot-1 female drinking the same amount as a 6-foot-4 male.

Their hydration needs would be completely different! There are two things I like to use to judge how much water to drink per day. The first is to go by how you feel.

Essentially, use your own internal thirst mechanism and drink water when you're actually thirsty. Your body will tell you when it needs more water.

When you're hydrated, you won't feel thirsty. Now, this may not be enough if you usually don't drink that much water.

That's why the other thing you need to do is judge your hydration by the color of your urine, like I talked about earlier. If your urine is a yellowish color, then you need to start drinking more water.

On the other hand, if your urine is clear, then you're hydrated and good to go. Doing this will help to keep things simple, and it'll be one less thing that you won't have to worry about tracking and measuring.

What Other Benefits Can I Get from Fasting Besides Weight Loss?

The one major benefit of doing intermittent fasting is that it's an easy way to help you burn fat. However, what are some other results that you can expect to see from doing fasting?

The first benefit is that fasting can improve cognitive brain function, which can help you with improving your concentration. Growing up in school, we were told to eat a big hearty breakfast in order to help us perform our best on a big test.

Think about this though—sometimes after eating a high-carb breakfast, have you ever felt sluggish at work or at school? It's not a coincidence as it turns out.

When we eat a heavy amount of carbs, this makes an amino acid called tryptophan more available to the brain. The tryptophan will then change into serotonin.

Serotonin is a neurotransmitter that is primarily responsible for creating feelings of happiness and comfort. The serotonin will eventually convert into melatonin.

You may have heard of melatonin before because it's a popular nighttime supplement that helps you sleep better. Of course, that may be helpful to you if you're taking it before bed.

However, getting extra melatonin from breakfast isn't something we want in the morning if we're trying to stay awake and focus on something! Therefore, by skipping breakfast, we can help to improve our concentration and productivity at work or school.

Another cool benefit is that fasting may be able to help you recover faster from sickness. Whenever you eat, your body has to focus some of its energy on digesting the food you just ate. Thus, by not eating anything, your body can save some of that energy and focus more of its attention on fighting the illness.

A third plus from fasting is that it will help you save two of your most valuable resources—time and money. Let's say you're eating 5-6 meals a day in an effort to lose weight.

This means that you have to spend more time shopping at the grocery store, preparing those meals, eating those meals, and cleaning up afterwards. That's going to eat up a huge chunk of your time, not to mention the extra money you'll have to spend buying that food.

Compare that to fasting, where you'll only be eating 2-3 meals per day. This involves less prep time, less time at the table eating, and less clean up.

You'll have more time to do whatever you enjoy the most. Not only that, but the extra effort you'll have to go through to eat more meals might make you more likely to quit on your diet plan.

The final benefit I want to talk about in regards to fasting is the fact that it allows you to fly under the radar. You'll still get to enjoy eating large sized meals, and people will start to wonder how it is that you're losing weight while eating these larger meals.

The reality is that you're skipping breakfast and saving those calories for later on, but nobody will see that. This is the way it should be.

You don't want to be that guy who says, "Sorry I can't eat that, I'm on a diet." And as long as you're properly measuring macros and using your 15% junk calories wisely, you shouldn't have to worry about uttering that phrase ever again.

I've Hit a Weight Loss Plateau, and I'm Not Losing Weight Anymore. What Should I Do?

Let's say you've been losing weight steadily, and then all of a sudden, you hit a wall. You've stopped losing weight at the pace you originally were.

What should you do? First, just take a deep breath.

As with any major endeavor in life, there will be obstacles that come up seemingly out of nowhere that must be overcome. You don't want to panic and drastically change your diet plan or anything like that.

Instead, the first thing you need to do is try to figure out why your progress has stalled. Go back and check your food logs, see if you've been doing anything different recently.

Have you been eating more calories than you usually do? If that checks out, then honestly assess how diligent you've been in tracking your calories and macros.

Have you been tracking every calorie that you've been eating and drinking? Have you been tracking it accurately?

Make sure you thoroughly check over the data first; the data, if recorded properly, doesn't lie. If you skip over the data and try to change something else, you could be addressing something that wasn't the problem to begin with.

Once you have thoroughly checked over everything, then you may need to adjust your caloric intake. For example, let's say when you first started, you weighed 250 pounds.

You'd figure out your caloric intake by taking 250, multiplying it by 13, and then subtracting 500 from that number. That would give you a total of 2,750 calories per day in this case.

Now let's say that you've lost 30 pounds and weight loss has stalled. It may be time to update your numbers.

What you'd do now is take your new bodyweight of 220 and multiply it by 13. Then take that number and subtract 500 from it.

This would now give you a total of 2,360 calories per day. If you feel that you're really close to reaching your goal bodyweight, then only subtract 250 from your calculated resting metabolic rate instead of 500.

This will have you losing half a pound a week instead of a pound. You'll also need to recalculate your new protein, carb, and fat intakes as well.

The macro percentages of 40% protein, 35% fat, and 25% carbs will always stay the same regardless of how many calories you're eating per day. Note that you only want to update your caloric needs when progress has halted.

If things are going great and you're losing weight, don't change your numbers. If it isn't broken, then don't try to fix it.

Is It Possible to Change Body Types?

The short answer to that is no, it's not possible to change your body type. If you're a true endomorph, you're not going to be able to transform yourself into an ectomorph.

You're not going to be able to change to a smaller bone structure or develop longer limbs like that of an ectomorph. However, with the proper lifestyle choices such as eating right and exercise, you can start to take on characteristics of another body type.

For example, you might be able to get lean enough to where you start to look more like a mesomorph rather than an endomorph. An ectomorph on the other hand, can build muscle and start to resemble a look more like a mesomorph.

You can also boost your metabolism to more closely resemble that of a mesomorph as well. Will your metabolism ever be as lightning fast as a true ectomorph, or will you burn off carbs as easily as an ectomorph?

Probably not, but that doesn't mean you can't improve your body's ability to use fat for fuel instead of carbs. Conversely, an ectomorph or mesomorph won't be able to match your potential for muscle and strength.

This is all about improving at the end of the day. Take what you've been given and make it better.

You're not in control of your genetics, so instead focus on what you are in control of. Keep in mind that the opposite of this can also be true.

For example, a mesomorph could start to resemble more of an endomorph body type through poor lifestyle choices. Maybe the mesomorph becomes sedentary and eats junk food all of the time.

Then a gut starts to form, and he's starting to look more like an endomorph. Even if someone is born with the awesome genetics of a mesomorph, it doesn't matter.

Regardless of who you are, dedicated effort still has to be put forth in order for you to reach your goals.

Can I Eat Snacks In Between Meals?

I'm not a big fan of snacking, and I haven't been for most of my life. It never made sense to me to eat a little snack that would rarely do anything to keep me full.

If I'm going to eat something, I want it to be a meal that can actually get me full instead of a little snack. Most of the time, snacking is bad for most people.

There are a couple of reasons for this. The first one is that you might not be snacking simply because you're hungry.

You could be snacking because you're bored and you want to distract yourself. Snacking because you're bored isn't a good way to pass the time—it's a good way to take you farther away from your goals!

Having specific times for when you'll eat your regular meals will ensure that you won't engage in mindless eating just because you're bored. If you find yourself tempted to snack because you're bored, find another way to distract yourself that doesn't involve eating extra calories.

The other reason why I'm not a fan of snacking is that most of the time, the foods you're eating aren't that healthy! Typically, people snack on foods like crackers, chips, cookies, candy, and other junk food.

These simple sugars and starches will provide you with no nutritional value, meaning they're empty calories. They won't fill you up at all, so you'll still end up eating just as much as you would during your regular meals.

And thanks to the spike in insulin, you'll also get to deal with blood sugar crashes and possible food cravings.

A lot of the time, snacking goes hand-in-hand with convenience. We grab whatever snacks are most accessible. This will usually involve some sort of pre packaged snack we buy at the store that isn't that healthy for us.

Or maybe we get some junk food from the vending machine during a break at work. The truth is that it's much more difficult to prepare a healthy snack ahead of the time.

Taking the time to prepare a healthier snack that might involve fruit, vegetables, almonds or some protein powder would be much better.

Even with that being the case, it's still better to skip snacks altogether.

Instead, save those calories for later on during your regular meals, and you'll get to enjoy eating more calories. It's that much less food you have to prepare, eat, and clean up, even if it is just a snack.

Conclusion

Thank you so much for reading this book all the way to the end! I hope this book changed the way you view losing weight.

At the end of the day, it all comes down to being able to do what's sustainable, staying diligent, and actually keep up with the plan. I created this endomorph diet in a way that will work with your body type, not against it, in order to help set you up for long-term success.

The rest is up to you. You now have a plan that will be able to guide you to where it is that you want to go; you just have to execute that plan.

Remember that we all have our challenges that we must face and overcome. Weight loss may have been something you've struggled with your whole life, but now you have the right information and the power to change that once and for all.

Yes, there are going to be adversities that you're going to have to overcome. Keep in mind though that there are some benefits to being an endomorph.

You're the strongest of the three body types, and you can build muscle the easiest. That's something ectomorphs wish they had an easier time with.

Focusing purely on your weaknesses and comparing yourself to others is only going to hurt you in the long run. Regardless of what body type you are, don't forget that no one is born with a healthy and fit body that maintains itself by doing nothing and eating junk food.

Whatever fitness goal it is that you want to achieve, you have to be willing to put in the work to be able to achieve it. With that being said, I wish you the best of luck on your fitness journey; I know you can do it!

Did you enjoy reading this book? If so, please consider leaving a review. Even just a few words would help others decide if the book is right for them.

Best regards and thanks in advance!—Thomas

Sources

(1) https://www.ncbi.nlm.nih.gov/pubmed/22825659

(2) https://www.ncbi.nlm.nih.gov/pmc/articles/PMC4853817/

(3) https://www.ncbi.nlm.nih.gov/pmc/articles/PMC5663956/

(4) https://www.ncbi.nlm.nih.gov/pubmed/19860889

(5) https://www.ncbi.nlm.nih.gov/pubmed/18282674

(6) https://www.ncbi.nlm.nih.gov/pubmed/8875519

(7) https://www.ncbi.nlm.nih.gov/pubmed/1765061

(8) https://www.ncbi.nlm.nih.gov/pmc/articles/PMC3838844/

(9) https://www.mayoclinic.org/healthy-lifestyle/weight-loss/expert-answers/vitamin-b12-injections/faq-20058145

(10) https://www.ncbi.nlm.nih.gov/pmc/articles/PMC3010674/

(11) https://www.ncbi.nlm.nih.gov/pmc/articles/PMC2958879/

(12) https://www.ncbi.nlm.nih.gov/pubmed/7369170

(13) https://www.sciencedirect.com/science/article/pii/S1871403X17300066

(14) https://www.ncbi.nlm.nih.gov/pubmed/7470437

Printed in Poland
by Amazon Fulfillment
Poland Sp. z o.o., Wrocław